AQUA FIT

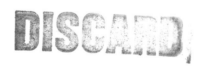

AQUA FIT

DR. JANE KATZ'S WATER WORKOUT PROGRAM

WITH YOGA, PILATES, TAI CHI, AND MORE

~ JANE KATZ ~

BROADWAY BOOKS

New York

BROADWAY

Broadway Books titles may be purchased for business or promotional use or for special sales. For information, please write to: Special Markets Department, Random House, Inc.

PRINTED IN THE UNITED STATES OF AMERICA

BROADWAY BOOKS and its logo, a letter B bisected on the diagonal, are trademarks of Random House, Inc.

Visit our website at www.broadwaybooks.com

First edition published 2003.

Book design by Tina Thompson
Illustrated by Jackie Aher

Library of Congress Cataloging-in-Publication Data
Katz, Jane.
    Aqua Fit : Dr. Jane Katz's water workout program with yoga, Pilates, tai chi, and more.
        p. cm.
    ISBN 0-7679-1482-1
    1. Aquatic exercises—Handbooks, manuals, etc. 2. Physical fitness—Handbooks, manuals, etc. I. Title.

GV838.53.E94K37 2003
613.7'16—dc21   2003040396

10 9 8 7 6 5 4 3 2 1

To my mother, Dorothea, who first introduced me to the wonders of the water.

And to water lovers everywhere, both the young and young at heart.

DISCLAIMER

Please check with your physician/health care professional before starting this or any exercise program.

ACKNOWLEDGMENTS

My many thanks to my editor, Trish Medved, and her assistant, Beth Datlowe, for leading the way and making *Aqua Fit* a reality. To Jackie Aher, illustrator, who has highlighted that a picture is worth a thousand words. And to Jason Guzman for his "icons" and charts. Thanks to the Broadway Books team, especially Gerry, Charlie, Rebecca, Umi, Elizabeth, and Chris, and particularly to Tina Thompson, for making this project float.

My appreciation to my family: especially my dad, Leon, who still shares the joys of water with us. To my siblings, Paul, Elaine, and June, and their children, Austen, Autumn, Stephen, Justin, and especially Jason, and Aunt Charlet, for her challenges in and out of the water. To Robert, Holly, Erica, Alex, Sidione, Dylan, and Tristan—for all their TLC.

More than ever in these challenging times, my thanks to my professional colleagues, John Jay College students, friends, swim buddies, and beyond. And special thanks to Emma. Hopefully the holistic benefits of water will be shared by everyone.

And finally to my best friend and cheerleader, my husband Herb.

See you in the water!

CONTENTS

PREFACE

In today's unpredictable world, it's difficult to take time out to relax, never mind to exercise. I designed the Aqua Fit program with this concern in mind, combining exercises that strengthen and stretch multiple muscle groups with aerobic activity and utilizing the relaxing, healing properties of water to create effective workouts for today's diverse lifestyles. With the holistic fitness that you obtain through Aqua Fit, you will feel more focused, energetic, and centered in your daily life and be able to accomplish more in less time. In other words, exercising with Aqua Fit will actually lead to more free time, something we can all fit into our schedules.

I began developing the Aqua Fit system long before I wrote this book. My technical knowledge of alignment and forms follows from over fifty years of experience as a competitive swimmer. I have taught swimming and water fitness in the City University of New York system for forty of those years. I became interested in sports medicine and water therapy following a crippling car accident in 1961. Through water rehabilitation, I was competing internationally just months after doctors told me that I'd never swim again. I also trained in the original Pilates studio before it was a household name. I grew up in what is now Chinatown in New York City, where tai chi was a daily community activity, and was exposed to variations of yoga body positions as a child gymnast. I learned the power of focused, controlled breathing as an elite swimmer and champion synchronized swimmer. With its combination of stretches, contours, poses, and attention to the breath, I often liken synchronized swimming to underwater yoga. As a result, I have always incorporated holistic practices into my aquatic fitness teaching.

Following the tragedy of September 11, 2001, I created a wellness spa at John Jay College in New York City to address the minds, bodies, and spirits of students, faculty, staff, and community members both on land and in the water. The spa included water exercise, Pilates, yoga, tai chi, soothing water music and nature sounds, chanting, candles, prayer, healthful food, and drinking water. Participants were able to regain some relaxation and peace during that tragic, chaotic period.

The success of the spa inspired me to create the Aqua Fit water workouts, bringing together yoga, Pilates, tai chi, and water exercise into a unique, comprehensive, effective, and enjoyable total water fitness program. Aqua Fit develops strength, endurance, flexibility, balance, and feelings of general well-being. It is designed to nurture mind, body, and spirit. So treat yourself to your own personal spa and take the plunge.

AQUA FIT

AQUA FIT EXERCISES

The Aqua Fit program consists of water yoga, Pilates, and tai chi exercises, as well as breathing, deep-water, and spa exercises. Each exercise includes a list of benefits and step-by-step how-to instructions. In addition, "icons" identify exercises that will improve strength, flexibility, balance, relaxation, or aerobic (cardiovascular) capacity. A list of specific types of athletes and other concerns for which exercise is prescribed (e.g., pregnancy) is also included. Finally, *Aqua Fit* contains a bonus family section to help prepare your infants, toddlers, and children for a lifetime of fun, safe water fitness.

Aqua Fit breathing exercises incorporate breathing techniques from yoga, Pilates, and swimming. Aqua Fit spa exercises are derived from yoga and the latest advances in water rehabilitation to provide the benefits of these exercises in addition to the healing properties of warm water. Aqua Fit deep-water exercises consist of deep-water running, treading, and jumping jacks for an intense aerobic workout.

Water yoga, tai chi, and Pilates are not simply land yoga, tai chi, and Pilates performed in a pool. They consist of exercises designed specifically for an aquatic environment and synchronized swimming figures that provide the benefits of land yoga, Pilates, and tai chi. I created these exercises through forty years of experience in synchronized swimming and water fitness and combined them for the first time in Aqua Fit. For years, I have likened many synchronized swimming figures to floating yoga postures and Pilates exercises. By including these synchronized swimming figures in Aqua Fit, I have put a new spin on land yoga and Pilates to give you a unique, superior workout.

There are many benefits of performing breathing, yoga, Pilates, tai chi, and running in an aquatic environment due to the attributes of water, including its buoyancy, resistance, density, and detoxifying properties.

Yoga, Pilates, and tai chi all consist of movements coordinated with breathing. The same holds true for aquatic exercise; thus, water is an ideal medium for breathing exercises as well as for coordinating movement with breath.

An important property of water is *buoyancy,* first discovered by Archimedes. Buoyancy is the upward force equal in magnitude to the weight of the water displaced by your body. This helps overcome the downward force of gravity. Therefore, your apparent weight is lowered in proportion to the amount of your immersion. Whereas running on land is high-impact and land yoga, tai chi, and Pilates are moderate-impact, all Aqua Fit exercises are low-impact. This means that Aqua Fit is much less stressful or jarring for your joints, muscles, and organs, making it ideal for both rehabilitating and preventing injury.

Buoyancy also adds a balance challenge to Aqua Fit because, as the extent of your immersion changes, you have to compensate for the changing contribution of buoyancy in overcoming gravity. As a result, the stabilization muscles that you use to balance are strengthened through Aqua Fit without the risk of falling that accompanies balancing postures and forms in land yoga and tai chi.

Due to the water's buoyancy, most of your energy in water is spent overcoming its *resistance,* which varies according to the speed that one moves through the water. Through Aqua Fit, you can further increase resistance by adding water toys (such as barbells, kickboards, noodles, and other equipment) that increase exertion. The muscle strengthening and toning provided by land running, yoga, tai chi, and Pilates are superior when done in the water.

Water is also denser than air, which is another reason that you float in water. Through floating, many horizontal Pilates and yoga exercises can be performed without the strain of the floor on your back.

Water is detoxifying. It has *diuretic* and *natriuretic* effects, causing your body to rid itself naturally of excess water and salt. Reducing water and salt in your body helps decrease joint stiffness. However, although your body will be cleansing itself through perspiration, you will never feel hot or sweaty, as you might during land exercise. The water's evaporation controls body temperature, producing a refreshing "air-conditioning" effect. This allows you to maintain your core body temperature and exercise for longer.

Water also provides *hydrostatic support*, constant, gentle pressure on every part of your body. This improves circulation by increasing pressure on the venous return (the veins returning blood to the heart) and strengthens the respiratory system by increasing pressure on the respiratory muscles. *(Remember always to check with your doctor before beginning this or any exercise program, particularly if you have a history of congestive heart failure.)*

A 2002 study from the American College of Sports Medicine revealed that water-based exercises are especially beneficial to those who find it difficult to exercise on land because of physical disabilities or embarrassment over their appearance, lack of coordination, and/or strength. The lucid cover of the water can help such individuals move more easily and feel more comfortable.

AQUA FIT WORKOUTS

The Aqua Fit program contains sample workouts designed to meet specific fitness needs and goals. Before you begin each workout, you may want to practice each exercise with a friend and the book on hand to ensure proper stance and movement. As you learn each exercise, you'll no longer need to look at the book. Each of the six Aqua Fit disciplines—water yoga, tai chi, and Pilates, as well as breathing, deep-water, and spa exercises—includes a sample workout that can help build proficiency with a particular type of exercise.

The remaining Aqua Fit workouts include exercises from all six disciplines. You can also choose from workouts for athletes, specific health concerns, flexibility, strength, and aerobic capacity to meet your individual fitness requirements. Additionally, the instructions for each individual Aqua Fit exercise include a list of benefits, which you can use to create your own unique workouts.

Each workout contains a warm-up, a main set, and a cool-down. Warm-ups are essential to raise your muscle temperature and get your blood flowing as well as to give your mind and body an opportunity to gear up, stretch, adjust to the water environment, and get ready for your main Aqua Fit set. They also prepare your joints and muscles to move more easily through their full range of motion. Cooling down and stretching out after your workout help you to relax, refocus, and bring your body back to its normal resting state. Gradually reducing your breathing rate and muscle temperature helps ensure a safe workout. For some Aqua Fit disciplines, specific warm-up and cool-down exercises are provided. In addition, energizing breathing exercises are wonderful warm-ups, while relaxing breathing exercises can be used to cool down. It's important never to skip your warm-up or cool-down, even if you are pressed for time. If you must shorten your workout, always shorten the main set rather than the warm-up or cool-down.

EFFECTIVE TRAINING

There are many goals of an effective workout, including building cardiovascular capacity, flexibility, strength, balance, and relaxation. Traditionally, fitness experts have measured the effectiveness of a workout by assessing aerobic activity through measuring the exerciser's heart rate. However, this measurement is relevant only for aerobic activity, which is just one method of increasing cardiovascular fitness. As discussed under the heading "A Holistic Program" (page 7), aerobic capacity can also be increased through slow, full breathing. In addition, heart rate does not measure whether a workout is effectively improving flexibility, strength, balance, or relaxation. In fact, an exerciser's heart rate may sometimes decrease as he or she becomes more relaxed, in which case an increased heart rate would indicate a *less* effective workout.

Despite these considerations, measuring heart rate is an effective way to monitor aerobic exercises. In addition, each person has a maximum heart rate that should not be exceeded for safety reasons. It is important to monitor your heart rate during exercise so that it does not surpass this value.

There are other tools that can be used in conjunction with heart rate to facilitate an effective workout, including the talk test, perceived exertion, and Aqua Fit training principles. The following section includes a discussion of each of these tools to help you plan your Aqua Fit program.

HEART RATE

Your heart rate or pulse is the number of times your heart beats per minute. It is one tool for measuring the effectiveness of an aerobic workout. To find your heart rate, take your pulse at either wrist or on either side of your neck at the carotid artery with your index finger. Count the number of beats for ten seconds and multiply that number of beats by 6.

Your resting heart rate is your pulse while you are sedentary. A lower resting heart rate frequently indicates greater cardiovascular capacity. Lowering your resting heart rate is one of the goals of exercising.

According to the American Heart Association and the American Medical Association, it is not safe for your pulse to exceed your maximum heart rate (MHR) during this or any exercise program. Your MHR is 220 minus your chronological age (220 – age = MHR). If you are thirty-five, your MHR is 185 beats per minute (bpm).

During an aerobic workout, your target heart rate (THR) is the ideal rate to which your workout should be geared. Your THR is 60–82 percent of MHR, depending on your fitness goals. To burn maximum fat, your THR is closer to 60 percent of your MHR. To build endurance, your THR is closer to 82 percent of your MHR. If you are thirty-five, your THR is 154 bpm for fat burning and 180 bpm for building endurance.

During the warm-up period, your pulse should gradually increase from your resting heart rate to your target heart rate. During the cool-down period, your pulse should gradually decrease from your target heart rate to your resting heart rate.

TALK TEST

Another method of measuring the aerobic effectiveness of your workout is by using the talk test. As I ask my students while teaching, "Can you babble while you bubble?" If you can carry on a partial conversation with your Aqua Fit buddy, you are probably exercising at your target heart rate. In this case, you would be able to speak two or three words, and then need to stop talking to catch your breath. If you cannot speak at all, you are probably overexerting yourself and should slow down. However, if you can carry on a full conversation with long phrases or sentences, you are probably exercising below your target heart rate.

PERCEIVED EXERTION

The concern of using both heart rate and the talk test is that they mainly measure aerobic effectiveness. Researchers in exercise physiology have found that exercisers themselves are best able to provide a guide to the effectiveness of their workout and how hard they are really working. Through estimating their perceived energy exertion on a scale of 1 to 10, exercisers can provide a guide to the effectiveness of many aspects of their workout, including increasing strength, flexibility, and aerobic capacity. Exercisers should strive for a perceived exertion target level of between 5 and 8.

Perceived exertion is even a good guide for aerobic effectiveness. During aerobic exercise, exercisers' heart rates rise in proportion to increases in their perceived exertion. Exercisers working below their target heart rate (based on pulse count) perceive that their energy exertion is light to moderate, or between 0 and 4. Exercisers working at their target heart rate perceive their exertion to be moderate to very hard, or between 5 and 8. As exercisers approach maximum heart rate, they perceive energy exertion to be very, very hard or maximum (9 or 10).

AQUA FIT TRAINING PRINCIPLES

Although the perceived energy exertion tool provides feedback about the effectiveness of a broader range of workout goals, it still provides no information regarding the goals of stress reduction and relaxation. During your Aqua Fit program, perceived relaxation is just as important as perceived exertion. You can use the Perceived Relaxation chart to think about stress reduction as a fitness goal. Try to increase your perceived relaxation both throughout a single workout and over a series of workouts.

The Aqua Fit training principles—frequency, intensity, and time—can help you increase perceived relaxation *and* work at a target level of perceived exertion. As all aspects of your holistic fitness increase, you can increase the frequency, intensity, and time of your Aqua Fit workouts by adding more workouts per week, trying challenging exercise variations, and increasing the length of your workout. Increasing the time of your workout can mean holding a balancing yoga pose or "asana" for longer, and increasing the frequency of your workout can mean adding more workouts per week. Therefore, the Aqua Fit training principles are a good gauge for measuring the effectiveness of all aspects of your workout.

PERCEIVED RELAXATION

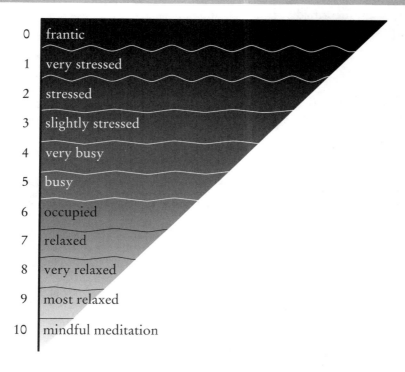

0	frantic
1	very stressed
2	stressed
3	slightly stressed
4	very busy
5	busy
6	occupied
7	relaxed
8	very relaxed
9	most relaxed
10	mindful meditation

A HOLISTIC PROGRAM

The Aqua Fit program is holistic. It benefits your entire person, supporting, balancing, and connecting your body, spirit, and mind.

BODY

The Aqua Fit program benefits your body through increasing aerobic capacity, flexibility, and muscle tone.

Stretching in water is easier and more effective than stretching on land because of the natural increases in range of motion and flexibility afforded by water. Due to water's resistance, any submerged movement strengthens and tones muscles. Drawing from the traditions of land yoga, Pilates, and tai chi, many Aqua Fit exercises simultaneously stretch and strengthen multiple muscles, helping you build total fitness quickly and efficiently. Throughout Aqua Fit, exercises that build flexibility and strength are identified with icons, and special Aqua Fit workouts for strength and flexibility include exercises from all six disciplines.

Aerobic capacity is the ability of your cardiovascular system to carry blood to working muscles, supplying them with oxygen from the air you breathe and carrying away carbon dioxide and other waste products. The greater your aerobic capacity, the less strain on your heart, the greater your ability to perform work and cope with stress, and the greater your feeling of well-being.

Aerobic activity is exercise that conditions the cardiovascular system (heart and lungs) by increasing the efficiency of oxygen intake by the body. Many Aqua Fit cross training and deep-water exercises and workouts are aerobic. Aerobic exercises in the water yoga, Pilates, tai chi, and spa sections are identified with an icon, and a special cardiovascular Aqua Fit workout contains aerobic exercises from all six Aqua Fit disciplines. The air-conditioning effect of water evaporating off the body prevents overheating. Therefore, you can engage in longer periods of aerobic exercise in water than are possible on land.

The Aqua Fit program also helps to focus on breathing. Deep, slow breathing helps air get into the deepest part of the lungs, where oxygen is separated from the air, released into the bloodstream, and combined with the hemoglobin of the red blood cells. When the concentration of oxygen in the blood is higher, the heart can beat slower and still circulate sufficient oxygen. In this manner, body cells receive life-giving oxygen and nutrients necessary to do the work of the cells and create energy, while aerobic capacity increases.

In a study at John Jay College of the City University of New York, the aerobic benefits of water exercise were compared to those of swimming. Aerobic fitness was measured by the important goal of a slower resting heart rate at the end of the program. Fifty-five participants, ages nineteen to thirty-five, were divided into two groups. One group participated in a twice-weekly water exercise program for eight weeks, and the other group participated in a traditional lap fitness program. The resting heart rates of participants in both groups decreased the same amount, indicating that water exercise provides the same benefits as traditional lap swimming, even for people with no swim ability.

Researchers from Temple University have also shown that working out in water is an effective exercise regimen. Twenty participants, all older adults, were divided into two groups. One group exercised in the water for forty minutes three days a week, while the other group remained inactive. After twelve weeks, those who exercised had improved their aerobic capacity by 15 percent over the group that had remained sedentary. This is called the "training effect," which helps condition the muscles to extract more oxygen.

SPIRIT

The Aqua Fit program is social and fun. It can be both relaxing and energizing, and it gives you a psychological boost. In addition, the Aqua Fit program will help you achieve a sense of well-being and balance in your everyday life.

Aqua Fit can be done alone or in a group. In a group situation, each person can design a unique program or use whichever workout suits his or her personal needs, enabling everyone to exercise with group support and encouragement without fostering competition.

In fact, if you have low energy, doing your Aqua Fit workouts with friends can be especially energizing. The divine buoyancy of the cool, refreshing water allows you to feel almost weightless and you can play upbeat, invigorating music. If you are feeling frazzled or anxious, you can play calming, peaceful music or sounds. While I am teaching water fitness, I incorporate everything from New Age and classical to jazz and rock music. Music can be an integral part of nurturing your spirit.

Water will nurture all of your senses. The sight, sound, touch, and smell of water are all soothing, and water tastes fresh and delicious! The natural increases in flexibility and range of motion afforded by water will help you to feel graceful and fluid. As soon as you are immersed in water, the day's tensions ebb away and you feel relaxed. Through the soothing power of gentle movement in warm water, the Aqua Fit spa exercises will help you feel more calm and peaceful. In addition, an icon identifies exercises that provide relaxation throughout *Aqua Fit,* and a special relaxation workout includes exercises from all six Aqua Fit disciplines.

During many Aqua Fit exercises, *endorphins* released by your body will give you a psychological boost and a feeling of relaxation. Endorphins are opiate-like hormones released during exertion that some experts believe are effective in fighting depression.

The Aqua Fit program provides both total tranquillity and vigorous exercise. Feeling this balance between relaxation and exertion will help you to create a life balance between work and leisure. This knowledge as well as the breathing, relaxation, and movement techniques that you'll learn through Aqua Fit will help you feel more confident that you can cope with life's challenges, even after you leave the pool.

MIND

The Aqua Fit program interacts with your nervous system to help reduce stress and improve focus.

Life can be stressful, and uncertainty about the future often leads to a great deal of anxiety and concern. We are hardwired to cope automatically with fear through a small nucleus, the *amygdala,* located near a part of the brain called the *thalamus.* The thalamus activates the sympathetic division of the autonomic nervous system, which enables us to respond appropriately to temporary emergencies by running away or defending ourselves (the fight-or-flight response). The sympathetic nervous system responds to fear by preparing our bodies. This results in sweating, rapid heart rate, rapid breathing, a rise in blood sugar, and shunting oxygenated blood to muscles to prepare us for action. When the temporary emergency or threat ends, the parasympathetic division of the autonomic nervous system restores us to calmness, slows our heart rate, and lowers our breathing rate.

However, in the case of more constant anxiety, the sympathetic division of the nervous system may be constantly aroused, and hormones like adrenaline can be increased. We can feel agitated or tense and our breathing and heart rates can remain elevated. This is referred to as stress, which can be very taxing on the body and bad for health. In this manner, emotions such as worry or apprehension actually lead to physical disease.

As we cannot control most of the events that occur in our lives, we must learn to relax and regulate the sympathetic nervous system so that we can focus on positive well-being and enjoy the moment.

Throughout the Aqua Fit program, consciously slowing your breathing can help counteract the increased breath rate caused by an overstimulated sympathetic nervous system. Regular exercise is also a vital part of keeping our body's reactions to stress in check. Often we hold stress in our bodies, which leads to knots, spasms, or muscles that are locked in tension. Endorphins released during exercise and movement help to relieve this tension. In addition, a regular exerciser's heart rate will return to normal faster than a sedentary person's heart rate after comparable exertion or stress.

During times of stress, our thoughts can feel out of our control and unfocused. In the traditions of tai chi and yoga, many Aqua Fit movements require balance, which results in concentration and attention to body position. The Aqua Fit focus on breath awareness also leads to focusing on sensations in your body instead of unproductive, self-defeating thoughts or stress in your life. Through both balancing and conscious breathing, you will bring your thoughts inward, center yourself, and create a mindful, meditative body awareness. Training your mind to focus in this manner will enable you to clear your head of cluttering thoughts and concentrate better in other situations. Even after you leave the pool, you will feel more focused and centered in your daily life.

GETTING STARTED

To facilitate safe, effective, and enjoyable Aqua Fit workouts, prepare for your program both physically and mentally. Gather any desired personal or aquatic equipment and take a moment to think about safety concerns and nutrition.

GEARING UP

The following are some suggestions to help you get mentally prepared for your workout.

Learn how to compartmentalize. Compartmentalization involves separating the different aspects of your life so that you don't become overwhelmed with work, school, or household and family responsibilities. Set aside time for your Aqua Fit program and commit to your scheduled program even if you are busy.

Direct your attentional focus. While you are in the water, try not to let distractions interfere with your workout; focus on the task at hand. Don't be discouraged if your mind wanders onto other aspects of your life, schedule, or responsibilities. As you inhale, congratulate yourself on noticing that your mind is wandering. As you exhale, visualize a bubble floating away with all of the thoughts that are cluttering your mind.

Maintain a positive attitude. Be proud of setting aside time to take care of yourself with your Aqua Fit program. Focus on enjoying your workout, not your fitness level, the fitness level of your Aqua Fit buddy, whether or not you are improving, or your shortcomings. Focus on how your body feels and moves, not the way your body looks.

EQUIPMENT

In order to physically prepare for your Aqua Fit program, gather some equipment that will enhance your comfort and enjoyment.

PERSONAL WATER GEAR

Swimsuit. Choose a bathing suit that is comfortable, lightweight, and becoming to your body. Be certain that there are no uncomfortable string or strap placements that can ride up or slip down and that your buttocks and bust are secure.

Lycra (spandex) is light, quick-drying, and very comfortable but will eventually develop threadbare areas at the hips, bust, or buttocks. The life of a nylon suit is longer, but many people find them less comfortable. There are also various combination fabrics available on the market. Whatever your suit is made of, be sure to wash it thoroughly after each use to prolong its life. Lycra bodysuits (like wet suits) are also available for greater protection outdoors and/or for warmth.

Waterproof watch. Give each Aqua Fit workout component its full, appropriate allotted time by wearing or having a watch nearby. When buying a watch to wear in the water, try on the watch and simulate some Aqua Fit exercises to see if the watch slips around your wrist.

Aqua shoes. Waterproof shoes, usually made of nylon mesh with a rubberlike sole, are helpful for cushioning feet during water exercise as well as for protecting feet and providing traction on a pool deck. They are recommended, and are particularly suitable for Aqua Fit exercises.

Head protection. If you're concerned about keeping your hair dry and protecting it, use a hair band with a Velcro closing or an exercise swim band. A swim cap will cover your hair fully if you plan to submerge your head. You can also wear a cap or visor during outdoor Aqua Fit workouts to help protect your face from the sun.

Goggles. Many Aqua Fit workouts can be done without submerging your face. However, if you wear contact lenses and/or you are combining your Aqua Fit workouts with swimming, goggles are recommended. (Prescription goggles are also available.)

AQUATIC EQUIPMENT

Many pools will have aquatic equipment poolside.

Kickboard. A kickboard is a flotation device that supports the upper body. It can also be used as a resistance device.

Hand paddles and gloves. Placed on your hands, they offer greater resistance to the water's surface. They're like fins for your hands. Mitts and gloves are also worn on the hands, with the larger surface area increasing resistance during arm motion and enhancing arm and shoulder movements, especially for tai chi.

Pull-buoy. A pull-buoy is a small float, usually made of Styrofoam. It can be used both as a flotation device and/or for resistance.

Fins. Fins are large paddles that are attached to the feet, used to increase resistance, and extend the foot. Fins have a large surface area, providing resistance to strengthen and stretch leg muscles. When used as extenders, the foot can be grabbed more easily. Finally, when used for water tai chi, they require a meditative focus on carefully and slowly picking the foot up off the pool floor for each step.

Cuffs. These are devices (sometimes inflatable) that can be placed on the arms or legs. They can be used as flotation devices for easy, relaxed floating and/or as a resistance device.

Flotation belts. Belts made of Styrofoam or other buoyant material keep the exerciser's head just above water. These are ideal for deep-water exercise.

Barbells. These are flotation devices shaped as the name implies. They are also available in molded plastic, which offers greatest resistance rather than buoyancy.

Noodles. These are also known as "logs." They are solid Styrofoam tubes, approximately five feet long and three inches in diameter. They are buoyant, flexible, versatile, and fun! They come in a variety of colors and can often be found in drug-stores and supermarkets.

AQUA FIT SAFETY

Although safety is always a priority, it is particularly important in the water, where minor accidents can have serious consequences. For this reason, you should *never* exercise in the water unless there is an individual trained in rescue breathing and cardiopulmonary resuscitation (CPR) present. You may want to contact your local American Red Cross or American Heart Association chapter to learn these skills yourself, especially if you own your own pool. In addition, get a medical checkup before beginning this or any exercise program, particularly if you have been sedentary for a long period of time.

Before entering the water, check for barriers, safety equipment, diving boards, water clarity, and lifeguards on duty. Read carefully any signage regarding water depth. In open areas, check for posted precautions, including water temperature, currents, tides, and submerged pilings. Never dive into unknown waters.

Next, you should start slowly and listen to your body. Always warm up before your main Aqua Fit set and cool down afterward. Breathe rhythmically throughout each exercise. Never hold your breath! Exhale fully during exertion to eliminate waste products such as lactic acid and carbon dioxide, and inhale during recovery. If any pain, shortness of breath, dizziness, or disorientation occurs during your workout, stop immediately, get out of the pool, tell the lifeguard or a friend, and rest.

Finally, if you are doing your Aqua Fit workouts outside, wear a hat or visor, sunglasses, and waterproof sunscreen. Sunglasses should have UVA and UVB protection. Sunscreen should contain PABA and have a high sun protection factor (SPF), 25 or over. If you are staying in the sun, reapply the sunscreen upon leaving the water.

NUTRITION

Nutrition and exercise are equal partners in the quest to increase health and fitness. Try to follow the Dietary Guidelines for Americans, listed on the following page, so that you have plenty of energy for your Aqua Fit workouts. See your health care provider/nutritionist for specific dietary concerns.

- Choose a variety of grains daily, especially whole grains.
- Choose a variety of fruits and vegetables daily.
- Choose a diet that is low in saturated fat and cholesterol and moderate in total fat.
- Choose beverages and foods to moderate your intake of sugars.
- Choose and prepare foods with less salt.
- Only drink alcoholic beverages in moderation.

You also may want to modify your eating schedule according to the time of day that you swim. If you work out before breakfast, have a light snack beforehand. If you work out at lunchtime, have either a midmorning snack or a substantial breakfast. If you work out before dinner, have either an afternoon snack or a more substantial breakfast and lunch. Finally, if you work out after the evening meal,

FOOD GUIDE PYRAMID

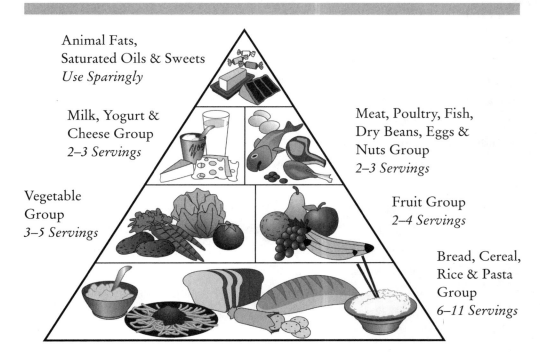

Animal Fats,
Saturated Oils & Sweets
Use Sparingly

Milk, Yogurt &
Cheese Group
2–3 Servings

Meat, Poultry, Fish,
Dry Beans, Eggs &
Nuts Group
2–3 Servings

Vegetable
Group
3–5 Servings

Fruit Group
2–4 Servings

Bread, Cereal,
Rice & Pasta
Group
6–11 Servings

have a more substantial breakfast and lunch so that the evening meal can be relatively light.

As you make your food choices and work out with Aqua Fit, try to aim for health and fitness rather than only weight loss. Weight loss, and exercise do not always go hand in hand. Overweight individuals who start an exercise program and also modify their diet will usually experience weight loss. However, participation in an exercise program alone can lead to greater cardiorespiratory and muscular fitness, as well as an improved sense of well-being and becoming fit, which are health benefits that are just as important as losing weight.

In addition, losing weight is not always an indicator of lower body fat percentage. At times, exercise may increase body weight at the same time as it decreases body fat, because muscle mass weighs more than fat. Therefore, you may look trimmer although you may not be experiencing weight loss.

HYDRATION

Drinking enough water is one of the best ways to improve your health. Water detoxifies the body, carries waste away from cells, dissolves many vitamins and minerals and carries them to cells, and regulates body temperature. Your brain, blood, and muscles are all made up of 75–80 percent water. Dehydration can lead to headaches, blood thickening, muscle cramps, and fatigue.

It is important to drink water throughout the day, because if you feel thirsty, you are already dehydrated. According to the Mayo Clinic, your water requirement in ounces is at least half of your weight in pounds. For example, if you weigh 160 pounds, you should drink at least 80 ounces or 10 cups of water a day, more during hot or humid weather. If you drink caffeine or alcohol, you also need more water. If you drink a cup of coffee or glass of wine, drink an extra cup of water at the same time. Finally, you need more water if you fly, because airplane air is very dry.

You also need to drink more water before, during, and after your Aqua Fit workouts, or any exercise program. Try drinking a cup of water within a half hour of beginning your workout, a half cup of water every fifteen minutes during your workout, and another cup within a half hour of finishing your workout. Even though you're going to be *in* water, you still need to *drink* water.

With dozens of brands of fortified water containing vitamins, minerals, and herbs appearing on grocers' shelves, staying hydrated during and after your Aqua Fit workout may seem complicated. Fortified water *can* be part of a healthy diet, but it often contains a lot of calories and costs more than regular water. Furthermore, if you are taking a multivitamin, it probably contains more of your vitamins and minerals than does fortified water. In most cases, regular, pure water is sufficient.

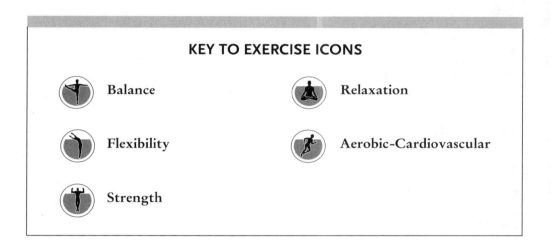

KEY TO EXERCISE ICONS

Balance

Flexibility

Strength

Relaxation

Aerobic-Cardiovascular

PART ONE

HOLISTIC WATER EXERCISES

Part One includes illustrations and descriptions of breathing, water yoga, water Pilates, water tai chi, and spa exercises. Each exercise includes a starting position and step-by-step how-to instructions as well as adjustments and challenge variations where appropriate. In addition, icons identify exercises that will improve strength, flexibility, balance, relaxation, or aerobic capacity. (See page 17 for a key to the icons.)

- *Breathing Exercises*
- *Water Yoga*
- *Water Pilates*
- *Water Tai Chi*
- *"Spaaah" Relaxation*

CHAPTER ONE

BREATHING EXERCISES

Breathing correctly during both your everyday life and your Aqua Fit workouts is essential for optimal functioning and health. Your goal should be to maximize each breath cycle by inhaling and exhaling fully in both the upper and lower lobes of your lungs. In the yogic tradition, this deep, slow breathing is called *pranayama*.

As you inhale, your abdomen and upper chest should stick out. This indicates filling of the upper lobes of your lungs through chest breathing and the lower lobes of your lungs through diaphragmatic breathing. Try not to lift your shoulders during inhalation, which is a sign of shallow breathing, using only the upper lobes of your lungs. Always inhale through your nose. The nostrils filter, moisten, and warm air, ridding it of dust and germs.

You can exhale through the nose, the mouth, or both the nose and mouth. However, it may be easier to exhale forcefully and completely through the mouth, especially during vigorous exercise. Complete exhalation is necessary to blow off maximum carbon dioxide and make room for inhaling more oxygen. During exhalation, your abdomen should flatten and your chest should fall.

Optimal posture helps contribute to correct breathing. Try to keep your chest open, your shoulders relaxed and not hunched, your upper back soft, and your chin neutral. Support your lower back by pulling your belly toward your spine. When standing, keep your pelvis neutral, not pitched forward, backward, or sideways. Maintain full contact between your feet and the floor and evenly distribute your body weight throughout both feet. This posture will enable you to fully inflate and deflate both lobes of your lungs.

It is important to think about breathing throughout your Aqua Fit workout. Holding your breath during exercise is a very common fitness error. In the traditions of land yoga, Pilates, and tai chi, throughout most Aqua Fit exercises movement is coordinated with breathing. This attention to breathing throughout your workouts will remind you of the guidelines for correct two-lobe breathing. In addition, breathing exercises are an opportunity to focus on correct, two-lobe breathing without any distractions. As you practice breathing correctly during your Aqua Fit workouts and breathing exercises, you will naturally begin to do so in your daily life.

According to Charles Stoebel, professor of psychiatry at the University of Connecticut Medical School, breathing can be implicated in 50 to 70 percent of diseases. When you are sick or perhaps stressed and out of harmony, you may find that the breath comes with difficulty, is more irregular, and comes from high in the chest, rather than involving the abdomen. The Aqua Fit focus on relaxed, full breathing can help prevent and even reverse the incorrect breathing that contributes to disease and discomfort.

Aqua Fit breathing exercises incorporate breathing techniques from yoga, Pilates, tai chi, and swimming. Special forms of breathing may alter blood chemistry and affect awareness or state of mind. Hence, certain Aqua Fit breathing exercises help to calm and relax, while others invigorate and energize. All deep and focused breathing increases our ability to concentrate and handle stress.

Each breathing exercise consists of guided movements and/or breathing to help center yourself and clear your mind. Except where noted, all Aqua Fit breathing exercises may be practiced standing in any depth of water as well as sitting on the pool edge or steps.

During each breathing exercise, bring your awareness to each inhalation and exhalation, thinking about correct two-lobe breathing. To help you focus, you can count your breaths or think of words such as "empty" and "full," similar to a balloon being inflated and deflated, with each breath. Alternatively, you can concentrate on your bodily sensations. As you inhale deeply, notice your chest rise and your abdomen expand. As you exhale fully, feel your abdomen flatten and your chest fall.

All of the Aqua Fit workouts in the remainder of this book contain breathing exercises. You can also use these exercises to rest during any other Aqua Fit workout. Finally, you can adapt any Aqua Fit breathing exercise to land to help cope with challenges in your daily life.

The following section contains how-to instructions for and benefits of the eight breathing exercises below as well as a ten-minute relaxing breath break and a ten-minute energizing breath break. Any Aqua Fit breathing exercise is suitable for athletes or those with injuries or special needs, except asthma. People with asthma should breathe at a natural tempo rather than impose patterns. Exercises that are safe for asthmatics and particularly helpful for specific groups are noted throughout this section.

Relaxing
- Calming Breath
- Rhythmic Breath
- Breath Retention
- Om Breath

Energizing
- Lion
- Breath of Fire
- Alternate-Nostril Breath
- The Hundred

CALMING BREATH

Relieves muscle tension

STEPS

1. Take a full breath, making your exhalation last for twice as long as your inhalation.
2. Take a normal breath.

AQUA FIT TIP ~ *You can try either Effleurage (in "Aqua Fit Pregnancy Prescriptive Workout," page 144) or Calming Breath while floating on your back. Wear a flotation belt, use noodles under knees, ankles, and neck, or use the corner of the pool for support as desired.*

RHYTHMIC BREATH

Relaxes

Rx: Asthma

STEPS

1. Practice this breathing exercise with or without face in water.
2. Inhale as you turn to one side.
3. Exhale as you return head to center, blowing bubbles if face is in water.
4. Repeat once.

AQUA FIT TIP ~ *Rhythmic Breath is a technique used for swimming the crawl stroke or freestyle.*

BREATH RETENTION

Increases lung capacity
Rx: All sports

STEPS

1. Inhale fully.
2. Hold breath for 2–3 seconds, focusing on the stillness in your body.
3. Exhale completely.

AQUA FIT TIP ~ *Breath Retention is a synchronized swimming breathing exercise used to increase lung capacity. Synchronized swimmers need to stay submerged for long periods of time.*

OM BREATH

Calms
Rx: Asthma

STEPS

1. As you inhale, bring hands to water surface, palms down, index fingers and thumbs touching.
2. Release breath slowly while saying "om." Empty your mind except for the sound you are emitting.
3. Inhale and exhale fully through the nose.

AQUA FIT TIP ~ *According to yogic philosophy, the sound "om" quiets and soothes the brain when said or heard. Also, "om" is the universal sound. If it were possible to hear either all of the noises in the universe at once or the vibrating of your chakras, both would sound like "om."*

LION

Helps with yawning and drowsiness
Rx: Asthma

STEPS

1. Inhale deeply.
2. Exhale with a roar, opening mouth, flexing hands, sticking out tongue, and arching back slightly.
3. Take a deep, full breath.
4. Repeat 5 times.

BREATH OF FIRE

Energizes

STEPS

1. Breathe in and out through the nose as quickly as you can while still using both chest and belly.
2. Place hands on belly to feel abdomen expand and contract with each breath. If you become dizzy or light-headed, stop immediately. This may occur if you use only the upper lobes of the lungs.
3. Repeat 10 times.
4. Take a deep, full breath.

ALTERNATE-NOSTRIL BREATH

Unblocks nostrils and eases breathing difficulties

Cleanses

Rx: Asthma, seniors

STEPS

1. Close one nostril with thumb or middle finger.
2. Take a full breath, exhaling and inhaling.
3. Close the other nostril with the thumb or middle finger.
4. Take a full breath, inhaling and exhaling.

THE HUNDRED

Warms up body in preparation for exercise

STARTING POSITION: Float on back with one noodle behind knees and another behind back and under each arm. Draw knees to body so that hips sink while calves remain at water surface.

STEPS

1. Inhale in five short bursts, contracting abdominals after each inhalation.
2. Exhale in five short bursts, contracting abdominals with each exhalation.
3. Pump arms about 6 inches with each breath.

RELAXING AQUA FIT BREATH BREAK

≈ 10 minutes	Calming Breath (8–10 times) Breath Retention (8–10 times) Rhythmic Breath (8–10 times) Om Breath (8–10 times)

ENERGIZING AQUA FIT BREATH BREAK

≈ 10 minutes	Breath of Fire (5–7 times) Lion (8–10 times) Alternate-Nostril Breath (8–10 times) The Hundred (once)

CHAPTER TWO

WATER YOGA

Yoga originated thousands of years ago in India but has become popular in the West only during the last few decades. "Yoga" is a Sanskrit word meaning "union"; it is often interpreted as union of the mind, body, and spirit or union of the physical self with the universal self. The ancient developers and practitioners of yoga, called *rishis,* were the first philosophers of India. They lived close to nature, so many *asanas* (yoga postures), such as Dog, Pigeon, Cat, and Eagle, are modeled on the movements of animals.

Asanas involve gently easing the body into increasingly challenging positions over time and through low-impact movements coordinated with breath. However, yoga is unique in that, depending on the asana and an individual's strengths and weaknesses, the challenge may come in the form of balance, flexibility, focus, relaxation, or strength. The world's strongest bodybuilder may be challenged by flexibility or balance, whereas the fastest runner may have little upper body strength and the most limber gymnast may find it difficult to relax and focus on breath. In this manner, each individual experiences yoga differently, works with his or her own strengths, and addresses his or her unique set of weaknesses.

Students of yoga report many benefits, including increased mobility and suppleness of the body, toned and strengthened muscles, the alleviation of postural problems, and in some cases weight loss. Beyond these physical benefits, they also report a sense of well-being, the ability to relax quickly and effectively, a focused mind, and in some cases a prevailing sense of inner peace and happiness.

Water yoga is designed specifically for an aquatic environment, to provide the benefits of land yoga asanas combined with the benefits of exercising in water. As mentioned in the Introduction, it includes some synchronized swimming figures, for which names of analogous land yoga asanas are provided. If you are not a strong swimmer or prefer not to get your head wet, you may wish to skip these exercises.

The following section includes starting positions, step-by-step how-to instructions, unique benefits, and variations of the thirteen water yoga asanas below as well as Sun Salutations and a thirty-minute workout. See the previous section for descriptions of the breathing exercises included in the water yoga workout.

Child's Pose is a relaxation asana that can be used throughout your Aqua Fit workouts if you need to take a break. Sun Salutations are a continuous series of asanas used to keep muscles pliable throughout your Aqua Fit workout and coordinate movement with breath. Water yoga practice always ends with three to seven minutes of Back Float, which is analogous to Relaxation Pose (shivasana) in land yoga. Although it is difficult for many people to take time out of a busy life to simply lie still, Back Float helps to cool down the body and cement the positive postural and alignment changes that are made during yoga practice. If you are very pressed for time, in just a few minutes you can squeeze in an Aqua Fit workout, recharge, and relax with five to seven Sun Salutations and three minutes of Back Float.

- Child's Pose
- Mountain
- Upward Dog
- Downward Dog
- Plank
- Aqua Lunge
- Warrior

- Toe Lock
- Cat
- Chest Expansion
- Shark Circle
- Water Wheel
- Back Float
- Sun Salutation

CHILD'S POSE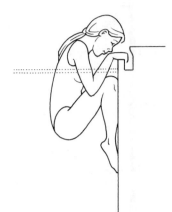

Relaxes entire body
Relieves tension in back, shoulders, and neck
Rx: Back concerns, sports

STARTING POSITION: Hold on to pool edge with bent elbows, shins on pool wall, knees bent, and toes pointed downward.

STEPS

1. Relax neck and let head drop forward or rest on hands.
2. Hold for as many breaths as needed to rest during Aqua Fit workouts.

ADJUSTMENT: Choose a knee position that is comfortable for you, anywhere from knees touching to shoulder width apart.

MOUNTAIN

Helps to open chest cavity and expand lungs
Stretches chest and abdominal muscles
Strengthens back, arms, legs, buttocks, and shoulders
Rx: Seniors, golf, running, bicycling, tennis, back concerns

STARTING POSITION: Stand with hands in prayer position in front of chest.

STEPS

1. Extend arms over head with palms pressed together.
2. Check your posture: back, neck, and chin should be in a straight line (no arched back or jutting chin); shoulders should be down and back; pelvis should be neutral; weight should be evenly distributed throughout both feet.
3. Focus on squeezing arms toward each other, trying to touch your ears with your inner arms.
4. Hold for 3–5 breaths.

ADJUSTMENT: Hold arms shoulder width apart or at another comfortable distance instead of touching palms.

CHALLENGE: While in Mountain, bend knees and squat as if sitting in a chair. Sit as low as comfortably possible. *Do not bend knees past a 90-degree angle.*

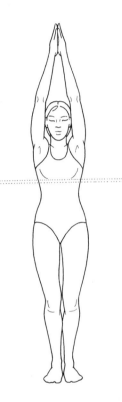

UPWARD DOG

Strengthens back, arms, and shoulders
Stretches chest and abdominal muscles
Invigorates and energizes
Rx: Golf, bicycling, back concerns, tennis

STARTING POSITION: Stand in waist-deep water. Begin by facing pool wall with bent elbows touching sides, toes touching the pool wall, hands holding pool edge, back straight, and chin near pool wall.

STEPS

1. Slowly inhale and straighten arms as you arch back to move upper body away from wall. *Be sure to use muscles of the torso, not arm strength, to arch the back, especially if you have back concerns.*
2. Push shoulders back and down.
3. Hold stretch for 3–5 breaths.
4. Exhale and bend arms, returning to starting position.
5. Repeat 3 times.

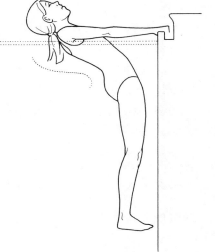

ADJUSTMENT: Instead of pool edge, use kickboard or noodle, which you can lower to the position under water that is most comfortable for you.

CHALLENGE: Use ladder or steps of pool instead of pool edge so that hands are lower and back arches more, or move feet farther from pool wall.

DOWNWARD DOG

Stretches back, hamstrings, calves, and shoulders
Strengthens back, abdominal muscles, chest, arms, and legs
Relieves lower back pain and tension
Rx: Back concerns, running, bicycling, tennis

STARTING POSITION: With both arms and legs bent, face pool wall, hold on to pool edge with both hands, and place toes against pool wall below hands.

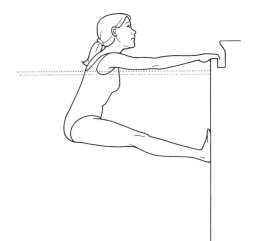

STEPS

1. Exhale slowly as you extend legs and arms into a piked position.
2. Place heels flat against the wall if possible.
3. Hold stretch for 3–5 breaths.
4. Inhale as you gradually return to starting position.
5. Repeat 3 times.

ADJUSTMENT: Begin in Child's Pose.

CHALLENGE: Hold stretch for 8–10 breaths. Rest and repeat 2 times.

PLANK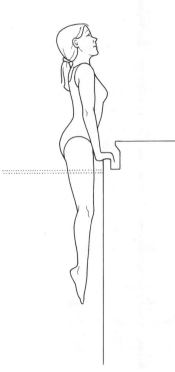

Strengthens upper body and abdominal muscles
Improves posture
Rx: Bicycling, mountain climbing, swimming

STARTING POSITION: Face pool wall with hands shoulder width apart on pool edge.

STEPS

1. As you exhale, bend knees, push off pool bottom, straighten elbows, and lift upper body out of water as if lifting yourself out of pool.
2. Inhale and exhale fully through nose.
3. Inhale as you return to starting position.
4. Repeat 7–9 times.

ADJUSTMENT: Stand arm's distance from pool wall with straight arms and palms on pool edge. Bring chest to the pool edge by bending your elbows as you exhale. Return to starting position by straightening arms as you inhale. Repeat 8–10 times.

CHALLENGE: Hold each push-up for 3–5 breaths and repeat 3 times.

AQUA LUNGE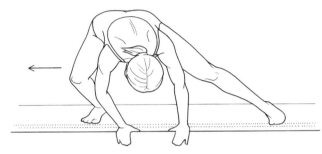

Stretches entire body
Strengthens arms and legs
Relieves stiffness in ribs and waist area
Rx: Pregnancy, golf, running, tennis, bicycling

STARTING POSITION: Face pool wall and grasp pool edge with both hands, shoulder width apart. Place feet against wall in a straddle position, beyond shoulder width apart.

STEPS

1. Shift body weight to right, bending right knee and keeping left leg extended.
2. Hold for 3–5 breaths.
3. Switch sides and repeat.

ADJUSTMENT: Stand with feet hip width apart in waist-deep water. Turn left foot out to approximately a 60-degree angle, keeping hips squared forward. Lunge forward approximately 5 feet with right foot, bending right knee so that right calf is perpendicular to pool bottom. Raise arms overhead, touching palms together and gazing upward at hands. Torso should be perpendicular to pool bottom and centered over hips. Hold for 3–5 breaths.

CHALLENGE: When weight is shifted to right, leave right hand on pool edge and create an arch by reaching overhead with left arm. When weight is shifted to left, reach overhead with right arm.

WARRIOR

Stretches entire body

Strengthens arms and legs

Relieves stiffness in ribs and waist area

Rx: Pregnancy, golf, running, tennis, bicycling, swimming

STARTING POSITION: Stand in waist-deep water with feet approximately 3–4 feet apart.

STEPS

1. Turn right foot 90 degrees to the right and left foot 30 degrees to the right while keeping hips squared forward.

2. Bend right leg until shin is at a 90-degree angle to pool bottom. Right thigh should approach parallel position to pool bottom.

3. Extend arms horizontally at shoulder level with palms facing downward and gaze at the middle finger of the right hand. Torso should remain centered over hips, vertical, and squared in the same direction as the hips.

(continues)

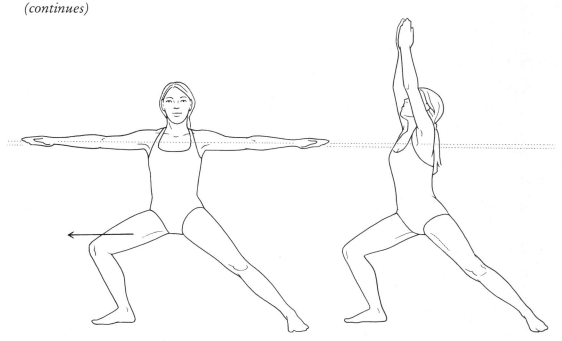

4. Hold for 3–5 breaths. Switch sides and repeat.

ADJUSTMENT: Reduce bend in knee. If additional balance is needed, place back against pool wall.

CHALLENGE: While in Warrior, square hips and torso in the direction of bent knee. Raise arms overhead with palms facing each other and gaze upward at fingertips.

TOE LOCK

Strengthens arms, legs, and abdominal muscles

Stretches arms, legs, and hips

Relieves stiffness in joints and muscles of the backs of legs

Rx: Golf, running, back concerns, bicycling, tennis, cross-country skiing

STARTING POSITION: Stand with back against pool wall.

STEPS

1. Hold right big toe with index and middle fingers of right hand.
2. Extend right leg as comfortably straight as possible.
3. Remain erect with correct posture. Do not bend forward at waist, round back, or lift shoulders.
4. Hold for 3–5 breaths.
5. Move leg as far as comfortably possible forward and return.
6. Hold for 3–5 breaths.
7. Release and lower leg.
8. Repeat on other side.

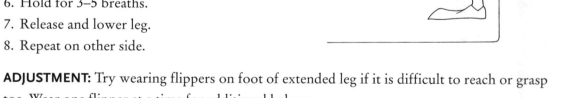

ADJUSTMENT: Try wearing flippers on foot of extended leg if it is difficult to reach or grasp toe. Wear one flipper at a time for additional balance.

CHALLENGE: Stand unsupported instead of with back against pool wall.

CAT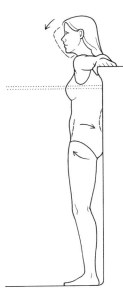

Strengthens pelvic floor muscles
Relaxes back, neck, and shoulders
Rx: Pregnancy, back concerns, seniors

STARTING POSITION: Start with back against pool wall.

STEPS

1. As you exhale, tilt pelvis upward by pressing small of back toward pool wall and look downward by bringing chin to chest.
2. As you inhale, tilt pelvis down and drop head back, stretching chest and arching back slightly.
3. Repeat 8–10 times.

ADJUSTMENT: Rest elbows on pool edge for support.

CHALLENGE: Hold tilted pelvis for 2 full breaths in each stage of Cat asana.

CHEST EXPANSION

Opens chest and expands lungs

Stretches shoulders, chest, and backs of legs

Rx: Back concerns, golf, tennis, running, bicycling

STARTING POSITION: Stand in waist-to-chest-deep water with feet together.

STEPS

1. Step forward 1–2 feet with right foot.
2. Bring palms together in prayer position behind back. Slide hands as far up back as comfortably possible.
3. Shoulder blades should be in line with back. Shoulders should be relaxed, not raised or tense. Hips should remain squared forward, as they were in starting position.
4. Hold for 8–10 breaths.
5. Release hands, step left foot forward to meet right foot, switch sides, and repeat.

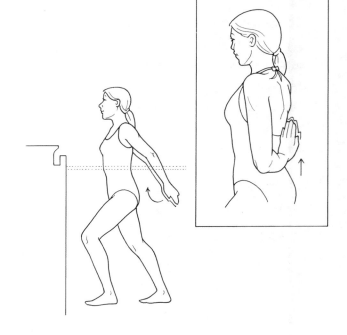

ADJUSTMENT: Bring palms together in prayer position at the small of the back or just touch your fingertips together.

CHALLENGE: Bend forward at the waist as far as comfortably possible while keeping hips squared forward and legs straight.

SHARK CIRCLE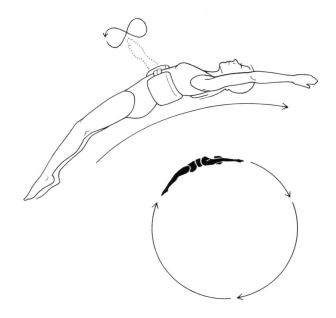

Improves respiration and posture

Strengthens entire body

Stretches abdominal muscles, chest, and thighs

Rx: Bicycling, running, skiing, tennis, swimming

STARTING POSTION: Float on back, using a flotation belt and a noodle between legs.

STEPS

1. Rotate onto right side with body arched, left arm extended overhead next to ear, and right arm sculling beneath hips to keep body afloat. Pressing left arm against head will cause head to submerge and help keep body at water surface.
2. Scull lower arm to move body in a complete circle following the body's arch. (See "Deep-Water Treading," page 100, for details on sculling.)
3. Return to back float and repeat on left side, sculling in a circle in reverse direction.
4. Repeat once on each side.

ADJUSTMENT: Stand in waist-deep water and grasp pool edge behind you with both arms straight. Tilt head back, contract back muscles, squeeze shoulder blades together, and shift hips forward to arch body. Relax arch before releasing pool edge. Repeat 2 times.

CHALLENGE: Don't use flotation belt or noodle.

AQUA FIT TIP – *Shark Circle is a synchronized swimming figure that provides the benefits of the land yoga asana Camel as well as the aerobic and strengthening benefits of continuous sculling and stabilizing your body perpendicular to the water surface.*

WATER WHEEL 🤸 🏋 🏃

Massages and cleanses internal organs
Stretches lower back and sides of torso
Strengthens lower back, hips, and legs
Rx: Golf, tennis, bicycling, skiing

STARTING POSITION: Float on back using a flotation belt.

STEPS

1. Scull with hands under hips to stay afloat.
   (See Treading in "Deep-Water Exercises" for
   details on sculling.)
2. Rotate hips 90 degrees clockwise while
   keeping upper torso flat.
3. Turn body in two complete circles at water's
   surface by alternately pedaling the legs.
4. Return to floating on back and repeat in other
   direction.

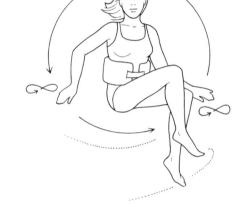

ADJUSTMENT: Wear a flotation belt.

CHALLENGE: Place right hand on right side of head and left hand on left hip. Use only the
pedaling of feet to stay afloat and turn body in circles.

> **AQUA FIT TIP** ~ *Water Wheel is a synchronized swimming figure that provides similar
> benefits of the land yoga asana Pelvic Twist or Spinal Twist without the strain of the floor
> on the back. In addition, it provides leg muscle strengthening and cardiovascular benefits
> of pedaling.*

BACK FLOAT

Relaxes entire body

Centers thoughts and breathing at the end of an Aqua Fit workout

STARTING POSITION: Use noodles under knees and behind neck. Alternatively, use pool corner, holding each edge with one arm for support.

STEPS

1. Lean backward, letting feet float off pool bottom, until you are floating on your back.
2. Relax forehead and let eyes close.
3. Release any tension in jaw and let lips part softly.
4. Relax shoulder blades into back.
5. Release any tension in neck, upper back, and lower back.
6. Let arms and legs be supported by noodles.
7. As you inhale, feel your entire chest and abdominal cavities being completely filled with air, bringing life and breath to your entire body.
8. As you exhale, release distracting thoughts and let the water rock away tension and stress.
9. Make a mental note of feelings of relaxation and contentment that you can bring to mind the next time you feel less than motivated for your Aqua Fit workout.

AQUA FIT TIP ~ *Back Float provides the benefits of the land yoga asana Relaxation Pose without the strain of the floor on your back.*

SUN SALUTATION

Warms up body before practice

Keeps body limber throughout practice

Stretches and strengthens entire body

STARTING POSITION: Stand facing pool wall in chest-deep water with hands in front of torso in prayer position.

STEPS

1. Inhale into Mountain asana.
2. Exhale into Plank.
3. Exhale into Upward dog.
4. Exhale into Plank.
5. Inhale into Mountain.
6. Exhale, moving hands into prayer position in front of torso.

Use adjustments and challenges from individual asanas as desired.

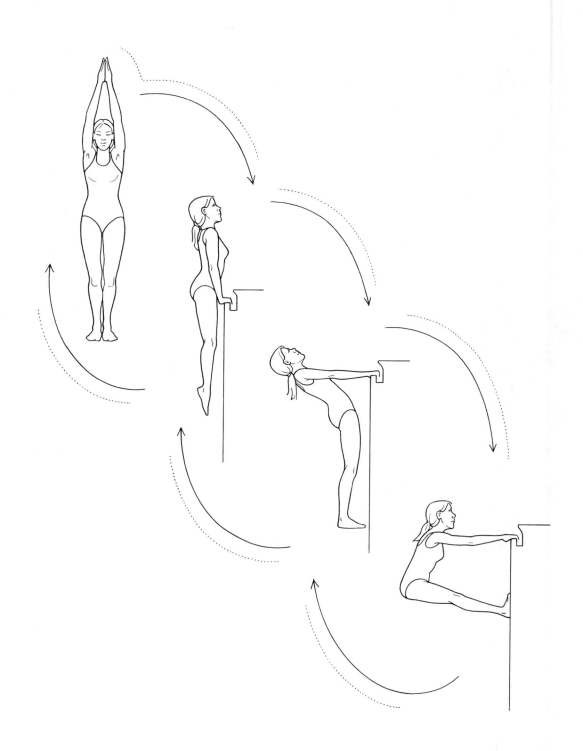

30-MINUTE AQUA FIT WATER YOGA WORKOUT

Warm-up ≈ **5 minutes**	Lion Breath of Fire

Water Yoga
Workout
≈ **20 minutes**
(2 minutes
for each)
	Asanas
	   Child's Pose
	   Mountain
	   Sun Salutation
	   Aqua Lunge
	   Sun Salutation
	   Warrior
	   Sun Salutation
	   Toe Lock
	   Sun Salutation
	   Cat
	   Sun Salutation
	   Chest Expansion
	   Sun Salutation
	   Shark Circle
	   Sun Salutation
	   Water Wheel
	   Child's Pose

Relaxation **3–7 minutes**	Back Float

CHAPTER THREE

WATER PILATES

As a child in Germany over a hundred years ago, Joseph Pilates suffered from asthma and rickets. He created a unique program of five hundred no-impact strengthening and stretching movements as a part of his own quest for health and fitness. Pilates movements are derived from yoga, modern dance, and gymnastics.

All Pilates exercises have fundamental principles in common. The breaths are full, producing muscle control without tension. There are no jerky, isolated movements. Every movement requires strength and concentration, with continued lengthening of the muscle. Integrated isolation focuses on stabilizing the area of the body in motion, but never isolating certain muscles and neglecting others. The body is seen as a comprehensive whole.

Pilates exercises are performed horizontal, most often while lying on the back. This makes Pilates ideal for people rehabilitating from illness or injury and others with limited mobility.

Pilates focuses on the torso, since all movements start here and flow to the extremities. This focus is based on the belief that most of our stresses and fatigue are the result of poor posture, imbalances in the body, and incorrect breathing patterns. The torso is instrumental in maintaining good posture and alignment. Strengthening and balancing the torso prepares the body for the rigors of daily life.

Pilates movements induce the heart to pump strongly and steadily. Blood is forced to carry and discharge accumulated waste products, and forceful exhalations remove these waste products. Regular Pilates practice is designed to strengthen and tone muscles, improve posture, provide flexibility and balance, and unite mind and body. Practitioners report a more streamlined body shape, suppleness, and grace, reflected in walking and movement. This is what makes it especially popular with actors and models.

Water Pilates is designed specifically for an aquatic environment to combine the benefits of land Pilates and exercising in water. As mentioned in the Introduction, it includes some synchronized swimming figures and unique Aqua Fit exercises, for which names of analogous land Pilates exercises are provided.

The following section includes starting positions, step-by-step how-to instructions, unique benefits, and variations of the twelve water Pilates exercises below as well as a thirty-minute workout. Water Pilates always begins with The Hundred breathing exercise (see "Breathing Exercises," page 21) to warm up the muscles and increase blood flow. Water Pilates always ends with Rolling Down the Wall, used to cool down the muscles and cement positive postural and alignment changes that are made during practice. You can also use Rolling Down the Wall as needed throughout your Aqua Fit workouts whenever you need a break. If you are very busy, you can recharge and relax in just a few minutes with The Hundred, your favorite water Pilates exercise, and Rolling Down the Wall.

- Leg Circles
- Ballet Legs
- Tub Turn
- Scissors
- Corkscrew
- Spinal Twist

- Leg Crossover
- Clam
- Mermaid/Merman
- Leg Kicks
- Single Leg Stretch
- Rolling Down the Wall

LEG CIRCLES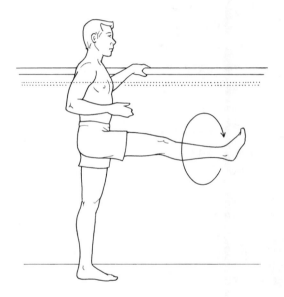

Strengthens legs, abdominal muscles, and sides of torso

Relieves stiffness in joints and muscles of legs

Rx: Seniors, bicycling, tennis, hurdles

STARTING POSITION: Stand in chest-deep water with left side next to pool wall, holding on to pool edge with left hand.

STEPS

1. Lift straight right leg 90 degrees.
2. Move leg in 5–7 counterclockwise circles.
3. Move leg in 5–7 clockwise circles.
4. Circles should be big enough so that big toe grazes pool wall.
5. Switch sides and repeat.

ADJUSTMENT: Lift leg forward 45 degrees instead of 90 degrees.

CHALLENGE: Wear a flotation cuff on ankle or try to balance without holding on to pool edge.

BALLET LEGS

Stretches back of legs

Strengthens abdominals, legs, arms, and shoulders

Rx: Tennis, bicycling, running, mountain climbing

STARTING POSITION: Begin by floating on back using flotation belt.

STEPS

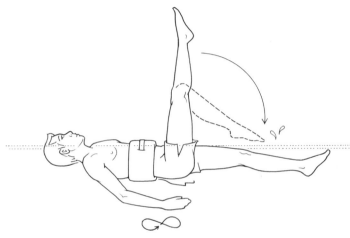

1. As you inhale, draw right leg up the inside of left leg by bending right knee until right thigh is perpendicular to water surface.
2. As you exhale, fully extend right leg in a slow, controlled motion, pointing right toes.
3. As you inhale, bend right knee so that right foot touches water surface, keeping right thigh perpendicular to water surface.
4. Return to floating on back while exhaling.
5. Repeat with left leg.
6. Scull with hands under hips throughout exercise to stay afloat and remain stationary.
7. Repeat once more with each leg.

ADJUSTMENT: Use a noodle under knee of leg that you are not bending and raising.

CHALLENGE: Practice without flotation belt.

AQUA FIT TIP ~ *Ballet Legs is a synchronized swimming figure that provides the benefits of the land Pilates exercise Single Straight Leg Stretch. It also provides the aerobic and strengthening benefits of using your arms to scull continuously, without the strain of the floor on your back.*

TUB TURN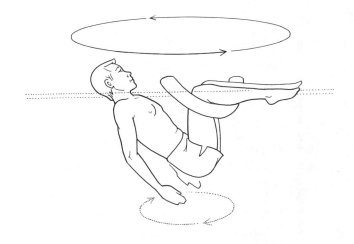

Stretches back

Strengthens abdominals, arms, and legs

Rx: Back concerns, bicycling, tennis

STARTING POSITION: Begin floating on back using flotation belt and noodle beneath knees.

STEPS

1. Bring knees toward your chest, keeping feet and legs together, until knees are bent 90 degrees, thighs are perpendicular to water surface, and shins are at water surface.

2. Remaining in the tuck position and keeping face above water, rotate body by sculling 360 degrees clockwise, pushing the water by turning palms sideways in the direction opposite to motion.

3. Maintain position and rotate 360 degrees counterclockwise.

4. Repeat once.

ADJUSTMENT: Add flotation noodle under knees.

CHALLENGE: Don't use flotation belt or noodle.

> **AQUA FIT TIP ~** *Tub Turn is a synchronized swimming figure that provides the benefits of the land Pilates exercise Double Leg Stretch as well as the aerobic and strengthening benefits of using your arms to circle continuously, without the strain of the floor on your back.*

SCISSORS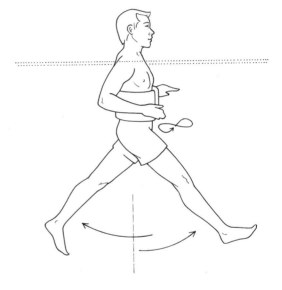

Stretches groin, hamstrings, calves, and quadriceps

Strengthens abdomen, lower back, hamstrings, and quadriceps

Rx: Running, bicycling, golf, tennis, cross-country skiing, hurdles, soccer kicks

STARTING POSITION: Assume a vertical position in deep water with legs together, wearing a flotation belt.

STEPS

1. Scull with arms to stay afloat.
2. While exhaling, move straight right leg forward and straight left leg backward as far as comfortably possible while maintaining correct posture.
3. Keep shoulders back and down and pelvis neutral.
4. Do not kick legs or make jerky movements; separate legs slowly.
5. While inhaling, return to starting position.
6. With next exhale, move straight left leg forward and straight right leg backward.
7. Return to starting position and repeat 8–10 times.

ADJUSTMENT: Hold a kickboard under each arm to stay afloat instead of sculling.

CHALLENGE: Don't wear a flotation belt if you are comfortable in deep water.

CORKSCREW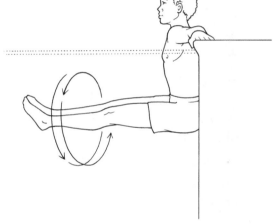

Strengthens abdominal muscles, hips, and thighs
Stretches thighs
Rx: Running, basketball, volleyball

STARTING POSITION: With back against pool wall, hold on to pool edge with both arms extended. Lift legs to a 90-degree angle, keeping them straight and creating an L with body.

STEPS

1. Circle legs counterclockwise: to the left, down, and back to starting position.
2. Inhale as you begin the circle and exhale as you finish the circle.
3. Repeat 8–10 times.
4. Circle legs clockwise: to the right, down, and back to starting position.
5. Repeat 8–10 times.
6. Keep entire back and shoulders flat against pool wall throughout exercise.

ADJUSTMENT: Lift legs 45 degrees instead of 90 degrees.

CHALLENGE: Hold a pull-buoy between your inner thighs as you circle your legs, and/or wear flotation cuffs on ankles.

AQUA FIT TIP ~ *Avoid this exercise if you have neck problems.*

SPINAL TWIST

Stretches sides of torso and pelvis
Strengthens sides of torso
Massages internal organs and improves digestion
Rx: Arthritis, golf, mountain climbing, downhill ski moguls

STARTING POSITION: With back against pool wall, hold on to pool edge with both arms extended. Lift legs to a 90-degree angle, keeping them straight and creating an L with body.

STEPS

1. As you exhale, pull with right arm, push with left arm, twist at the waist, and swing your legs as far as comfortably possible to the right.
2. Inhale as you return to starting position.
3. As you exhale, pull with left arm and push with right arm to swing your legs left.
4. Inhale as you return to starting position.
5. Your upper back and shoulders should remain flat against pool wall.
6. Repeat 5–8 times.

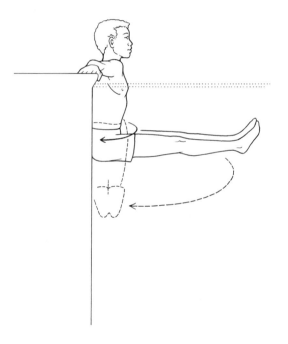

ADJUSTMENT: Lift legs 45 degrees instead of 90 degrees. Use corner of pool for extra support for back, shoulders, and neck.

CHALLENGE: Repeat 10–15 times.

LEG CROSSOVER

Stretches lower and middle back, hamstrings, inner thighs, and calves

Strengthens abdominal muscles, inner and outer thighs

Relieves stiffness in groin

Rx: Tennis

STARTING POSITION: With back against pool wall, hold on to pool edge with both arms extended. Lift your legs to a 90-degree angle, keeping them straight and creating an L with body.

STEPS

1. Separate your legs into a V, then bring them back together.
2. Alternately open and close your legs, maintaining the 90-degree L and keeping your legs straight.
3. Breathe deeply and repeat this opening/closing motion for 1–1½ minutes.

(continues)

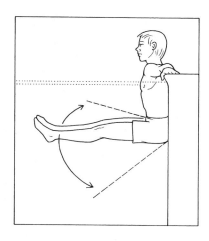
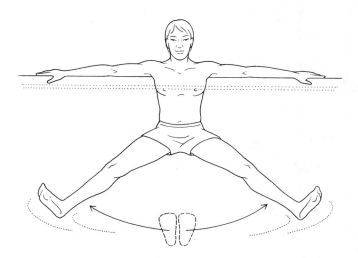

ADJUSTMENT: Lift legs 45 degrees instead of 90 degrees. Use corner of pool for extra back and neck support.

CHALLENGE: Begin by opening legs as far as possible. Keeping left leg stationary, bring right leg completely over to meet left leg. Return to open position and repeat with other leg. Breathe deeply and repeat these motions for 2 minutes.

> **AQUA FIT TIP** ~ *Leg Crossover provides the benefits of the land Pilates exercises Inner Thigh Lifts and Side Kicks Up/Down in addition to strengthening abdominal muscles.*

CLAM

Strengthens abdominal muscles, arms, shoulders, hips, and legs
Stretches backs of legs and entire back
Rx: Running, tennis, golf

STARTING POSITION: Begin floating on back in chest-deep water with arms extended overhead.

STEPS

1. Exhale as you pike hips down, raise straight legs to chest, reach for feet with straight arms.
2. Only bring hands and feet as close together as comfortably possible without rounding back or shoulders.
3. Return to starting position and inhale.
4. Repeat 8–10 times.

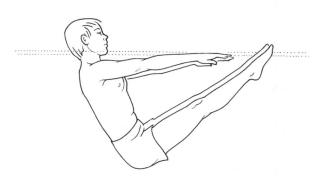

ADJUSTMENT: Practice movement with heels on pool edge and/or with a noodle under arms.

CHALLENGE: Bring hands and feet closer together and submerge body, exhaling through nose and mouth, forming bubbles.

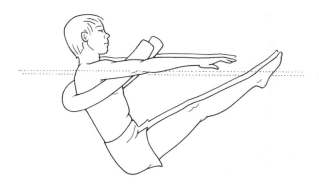

AQUA FIT TIP ~ *The "Clam" is also a synchronized swimming figure that provides the benefits of the land Pilates exercise The Teaser without the pressure of the floor on your tailbone. Your body will submerge with each repetition, reminding you to focus on your breathing, exhale during exertion underwater, and inhale during recovery above water.*

MERMAID/MERMAN

Energizes and invigorates

Helps to open chest cavity and expand lungs

Strengthens and stretches sides of torso and arms

Rx: Golf, running, bicycling, tennis, swimming

STARTING POSITION: Stand with feet together in chest-deep water and left side less than an arm's length away from pool wall.

STEPS

1. Hold pool edge with left hand and raise right arm overhead.
2. Exhale as you move hips to right, pulling on pool edge with body weight and keeping upper body in same plane as legs.
3. Create a smooth arc with entire right side of body by reaching with raised right arm.
4. Hold for 8–10 breaths.
5. Return body to vertical position before releasing pool edge.
6. Switch sides and repeat.

ADJUSTMENT: Stand a full arm's length away from pool wall.

CHALLENGE: Stand with edge of inside foot touching pool wall or at any closer comfortable distance away from pool wall.

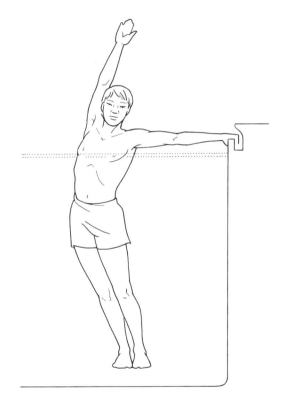

LEG KICKS

Stretches quadriceps
Strengthens thighs, buttocks, and lower back
Rx: Golf, soccer kicks, hurdles

STARTING POSITION: Face pool wall in deep water and support body with both forearms on pool edge. Do not hoist body out of water or lean body on pool edge. Keep shoulders down and back and neck in line with spine.

STEPS

1. As you exhale, bring feet to buttocks by bending knees.
2. Don't jerk feet toward buttocks; lift them slowly and squeeze them toward buttocks.
3. As you inhale, lower feet to starting position.
4. Repeat 16–20 times.

ADJUSTMENT: Bend knees to 90 degrees.

CHALLENGE: Hold a pull-buoy between inner thighs and focus on squeezing legs together throughout exercise. Wear fins on both feet.

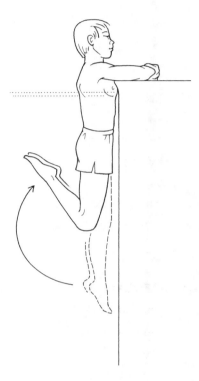

SINGLE LEG STRETCH

Strengthens abdominals and legs

Helps to relieve lower back concerns

Rx: Back concerns, seniors

STARTING POSITION: Stand in chest-deep water, with your back against the pool wall.

STEPS

1. Inhale as you grasp right knee and bring it toward your chest.
2. Hold for 3–4 breaths.
3. As you exhale, release and straighten leg.
4. Hold leg as high as comfortable for 3–4 breaths.
5. Exhale and return to starting position.
6. Repeat with other leg.

ADJUSTMENT: Hold on to the pool edge for support.

CHALLENGE: Pull knee toward chest as high as possible, then straighten leg close to the water's surface before returning to the starting position.

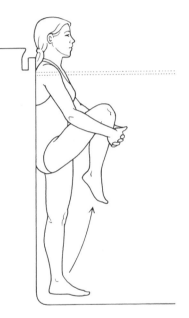

ROLLING DOWN THE WALL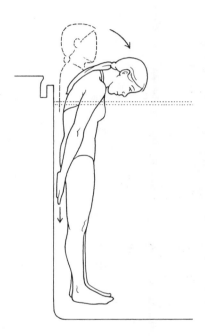

Relaxes entire body

Centers thoughts and breathing at the end of an Aqua Fit workout

STARTING POSITION: Stand with back against pool wall and feet approximately 8–10 inches from wall in chest-deep water.

STEPS

1. Beginning by lowering chin to chest, roll down pool wall as slowly as possible by removing one vertebra at a time from pool wall to create a perfect curve with spine.
2. Pull abdominal muscles inward to support lower back.
3. Only roll down to a point at which tailbone maintains contact with pool wall.
4. Let your neck relax and your head and arms hang.
5. Take five full, deep breaths.
6. Roll back up pool wall to starting position one vertebra at a time, as slowly as possible.

30-MINUTE AQUA FIT WATER PILATES WORKOUT

Warm-up ≈ **5 minutes**	Alternate-Nostril Breath The Hundred
Water Pilates Workout ≈ **20 minutes** (**1½ minutes** **each**)	Exercises *Leg Circles* *Ballet Legs* *Tub Turn* *Scissors* *Corkscrew* *Spinal Twist* *Leg Crossover* *Clam* *Mermaid/Merman* *Leg Kicks* *Single Leg Stretch*
Relaxation ≈ **5 minutes**	Rolling Down the Wall Om Breath

CHAPTER FOUR

WATER TAI CHI

Tai chi originated in the eighteenth and nineteenth centuries in China to promote health and self-defense. Each household had its own unique form that was passed down from one generation to the next. *Tai chi ch'uan* translates as "the supreme ultimate fist" or "the way of supreme harmony."

The Chinese believe that the life force or *chi* flows through all of us. Human beings have seven chakras or energy centers in their bodies. Daily stressors unbalance chakras and block the flow of chi through our bodies. Tai chi allows the body to open up, the muscles to relax, the tissues to expand, and the joints to open and connect, so that chakras are balanced and chi can flow more freely through the body. Water is an ideal medium for tai chi because it is inherently balancing for chakras.

Once this starts to happen, you feel greatly energized and it becomes increasingly easier to relax. As energy starts to move more freely, it accumulates in the *dantian,* an area of the body centered approximately two inches below the navel and a third of the way into the body. The dantian acts as a central storage area for chi. This generation and collection of chi is why tai chi is known for increasing energy and stamina.

Tai chi consists of slow, soft, relaxed movements or *forms.* One form flows into the next without pauses. The attention stays focused on every movement. Movements of the head, body, arms, hands, legs, feet, and eyes are coordinated, and all movement originates in the dantian. All forms have a yin or yang quality and contain aspects of both. The *yin* aspects and forms are those that contract, sink, or move inward. The *yang* forms and aspects are those that expand, rise, or move outward. Yin will always turn into yang and vice versa; this is how the forms "breathe." Inhalation occurs during the yin stages and exhalation during the yang stages.

Water tai chi consists of exercises that incorporate many movements and concepts from land tai chi. In fact, through learning Aqua Fit water tai chi, you'll acquire many skills that will be helpful if you decide to learn a full land tai chi form. If you already practice advanced land tai chi, water tai chi is a great opportunity to review basic skills and improve your form.

The most challenging aspect of both water tai chi and land tai chi is mental, not physical. Tai chi is a form of meditation, and it is difficult to constantly focus on the breath and such small, specific movements. Don't be discouraged if you find your mind wandering throughout the exercises. It takes time and practice to train your mind to center on bodily sensations instead of distracting thoughts. However, as you learn to concentrate in this manner, you will notice changes in your daily life. It will be easier to concentrate, as well as manage stress, frustrations, and regrets.

The following section contains step-by-step how-to instructions and benefits for the water tai chi exercises. You can practice water tai chi exercises in any depth of water. Choose deeper water for a challenging variation and shallow water for less resistance. The instructions for each motion are divided into steps to provide clear, detailed directions. However, as with land tai chi, each water tai chi exercise should consist of continuous, breath-coordinated movement. The body parts in motion should move smoothly, without pauses or accelerations.

- Tai Chi Walk Forward
- Tai Chi Walk Backward
- Tai Chi Opening
- Circle Water Spray Right
- Circle Water Spray Left
- Roll the Ball
- Hands Like Clouds
- Yin Yang
- Full Moon
- Tai Chi Closing

TAI CHI WALK FORWARD 🤸 🏋 🧘

Stretches ankles
Strengthens ankles and legs
Rx: Seniors, golf, tennis

STARTING POSITION: Stand with left leg forward, feet flat on pool bottom, hands on hips, and weight on left foot. Use a small scull at the hips for added balance.

STEPS

1. As you inhale, lift right heel, lift and flex right toes, and extend right leg straight forward, brushing pool bottom next to left foot with ball of right foot.
2. As you exhale, touch pool bottom with right heel, lower right toes, and shift weight to right foot.
3. As you inhale, lift left heel, lift and flex left toes, and extend left leg straight forward, brushing pool bottom next to right foot with ball of left foot.
4. As you exhale, touch pool bottom with left heel, lower left toes, and shift weight to left foot, returning to starting position.
5. Repeat 10 times.

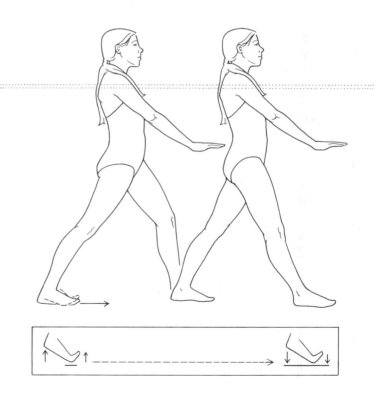

TAI CHI WALK BACKWARD

Stretches ankles
Strengthens ankles and legs
Rx: Seniors, golf, tennis

STARTING POSITION: Stand with left leg forward, feet flat on pool bottom, hands on hips, and weight on right foot. Use a small scull at the hips for added balance.

STEPS

1. As you inhale, lift and flex left toes, lift left heel, and extend left leg backward, brushing pool bottom next to right foot with ball of left foot.

2. As you exhale, touch pool bottom with left toes, lower left heel, and shift weight to left foot.

3. As you inhale, lift and flex right toes, lift right heel, and extend right leg backward, brushing pool bottom next to left foot with heel of right foot.

4. As you exhale, touch pool bottom with right toes, lower right heel, and shift weight to right foot, returning to starting position.

5. Repeat 10 times.

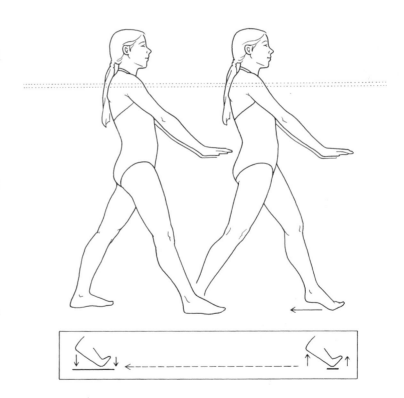

TAI CHI OPENING 🤸 🏋 🧘

Strengthens and stretches entire body
Rx: Seniors, tennis, golf, running, swimming

STARTING POSITION: Stand with feet shoulder width apart and arms at sides.

STEPS

1. As you inhale, raise both arms straight until hands are at chest level.
2. As you exhale, draw elbow to waist and bend arms until forearms are parallel to water surface. Keep forearms parallel to each other and palms facing downward.
3. As you inhale, bring hands to hip level by straightening arms while keeping elbows in place.
4. As you exhale, flex wrists slightly until palms are parallel to water surface.
5. Repeat 5–7 times.

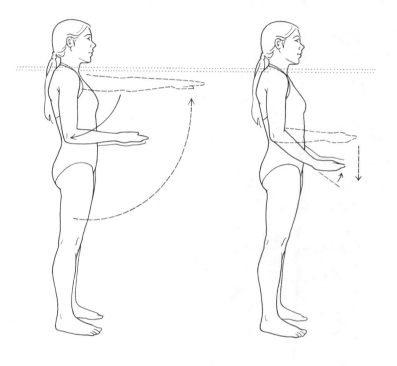

CHALLENGE: As you become more familiar with these movements, perform steps 1 and 2 during inhalation and steps 3 and 4 during exhalation. Repeat 10–12 times.

CIRCLE WATER SPRAY RIGHT

Stretches sides of torso, ankles, buttocks, and hips

Strengthens entire body

Rx: Seniors

STARTING POSITION: Stand with feet hip width apart, straight arms extended at sides, hands at water surface, weight on left foot, and tips of fingers submerged.

STEPS

1. As you inhale, pick up right toes, pivot right foot 90 degrees on right heel, and put down right toes. Keep hips and torso squared forward as they were in starting position.

2. As you exhale, shift weight to right foot, pick up left heel, and pivot 90 degrees on left toes, so that entire body rotates 90 degrees to right. Fingers move through water in a quarter circle and spray water as torso rotates.

3. As you inhale, lift left toes and bend left knee so that left thigh is perpendicular to torso.

4. As you exhale, place left toes on pool bottom so that feet are shoulder width apart, put down left heel, and shift weight onto left foot.

> **AQUA FIT TIP** ~ *After completing Circle Water Spray Right, you will have returned to starting position and rotated 90 degrees. You can stop there or repeat three times to complete a Full Circle Water Spray and experience a longer period of slow, constant, breath-coordinated movement, as you would in a continuous tai chi form.*

CIRCLE WATER SPRAY LEFT

Stretches sides of torso
Strengthens entire body
Rx: Seniors

STARTING POSITION: Stand with feet hip width apart, straight arms extended at sides, hands at water surface, weight on right foot, and tips of fingers submerged.

STEPS

1. As you inhale, pick up left toes, pivot left foot 90 degrees on left heel, and put down left toes. Keep hips and torso squared forward as they were in starting position. *(continues)*

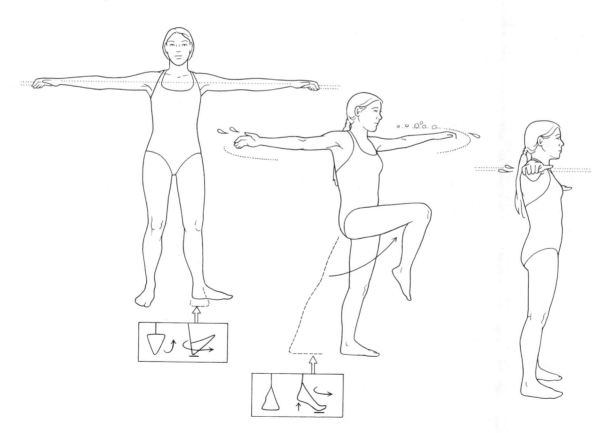

2. As you exhale, shift weight to left foot, pick up right heel, and pivot 90 degrees on right toes, so that entire body rotates 90 degrees to left. Fingers move through water in a quarter circle and spray water as torso rotates.

3. As you inhale, lift right toes and bend right knee so that right thigh is perpendicular to torso.

4. As you exhale, place right toes on pool bottom so that feet are shoulder width apart, put down right heel, and shift weight onto right foot.

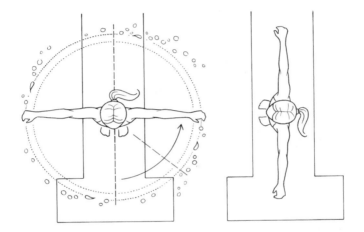

ROLL THE BALL

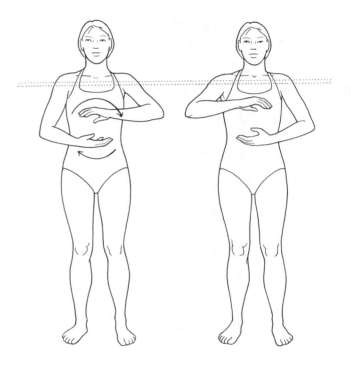

Stretches and strengthens arms, wrists, and shoulders

Rx: Seniors, tennis, boxing punches

STARTING POSITION: Hold left hand palm down at chest level and right hand palm up at waist level, with both arms slightly bent, as if holding a ball. Fingers should be slightly bent and spread.

STEPS

1. As you inhale, turn the imaginary ball over so that your right hand is palm down at chest level and left hand is palm up at waist level.
2. As you exhale, turn the imaginary ball back the other way.
3. Repeat 16–20 times.

HANDS LIKE CLOUDS

Stretches and strengthens arms, wrists, and shoulders

Rx: Pregnancy, seniors, golf, tennis

STARTING POSITION: To the right of torso, hold left hand palm down at chest level and right hand palm up at waist level, with both arms slightly bent, as if holding a ball. Fingers should be slightly bent and spread.

STEPS

1. As you inhale, rotate left palm 90 degrees, so that it is facing away from body instead of down as you move left hand as far left as possible without straightening wrist or elbow. Next, rotate left hand 180 degrees so that palm is facing upward at waist level as if

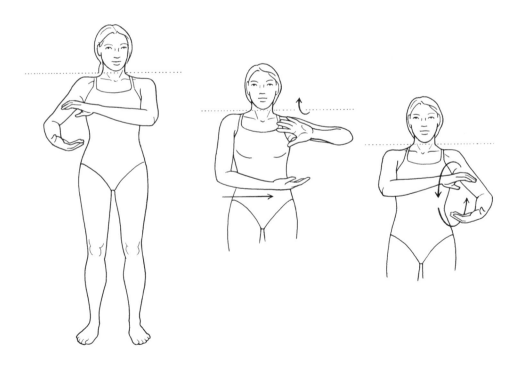

rubbing the surface of a larger imaginary ball. *Simultaneously,* move right hand left to just beyond torso. Next, rotate right hand 180 degrees so that palm is facing downward at chest level as if you are rubbing the surface of an imaginary ball. Palms should be facing each other to the left of the torso.

2. As you exhale, move hands laterally to right of torso. Rotate right palm 90 degrees, so that it is facing away from body instead of down as you move right hand as far right as possible without straightening wrist or elbow. Next, rotate right hand 180 degrees so that palm is facing upward at waist level as if rubbing the surface of a larger imaginary ball. *Simultaneously,* move left hand right to just beyond torso. Next, rotate left hand 180 degrees so that palm is facing downward at chest level as if you are rubbing the surface of an imaginary ball. Palms should be facing each other to the right of torso as in starting position.

3. Repeat 8–10 times.

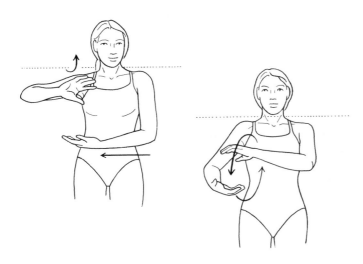

YIN YANG

Stretches shoulders, forearms, and wrists

Strengthens arms and shoulders

Helps with repetitive stress injuries from keyboard tasks

Rx: Seniors, golf, tennis

STARTING POSITION: Stand with hands in prayer position in front of chest.

STEPS

1. Keeping hands together, rotate hands 90 degrees so that right palm faces body and left palm faces away from body.
2. As you exhale, straighten arms by pushing right palm away from body with left palm.
3. As you inhale, push left palm back toward body with right palm.
4. Rotate hands 180 degrees so that left palm faces body and right palm faces away from body.
5. As you exhale, straighten arms by pushing left palm away from body with right palm.
6. As you inhale, push right palm back toward body with left palm.
7. Repeat 5–7 times.

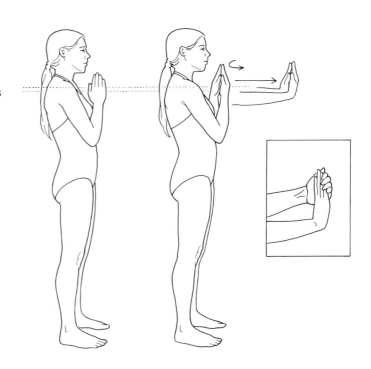

FULL MOON

Stretches and strengthens shoulders and arms

Rx: Pregnancy, golf, tennis

STARTING POSITION: Stand with feet hip width apart and hands at sides.

STEPS

1. As you inhale, lift arms overhead by moving them in parallel 180-degree arcs in front of body.
2. As you exhale, lower arms to sides by moving them in complementary 180-degree arcs at sides of body.
3. Repeat 8–10 times.

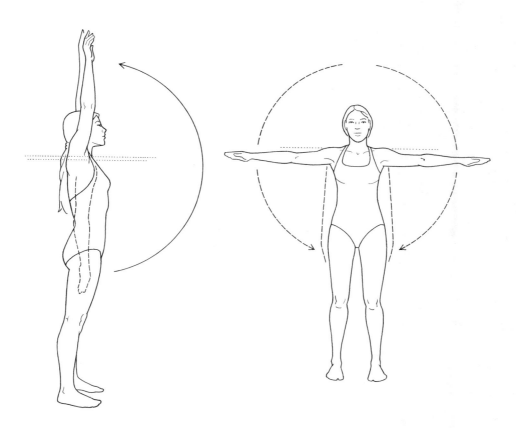

TAI CHI CLOSING

Strengthens and stretches entire body

Rx: Seniors, golf

STARTING POSITION: Stand with feet approximately 2 feet apart, legs slightly bent, arms at sides, and palms facing backward.

STEPS

1. As you inhale, rotate palms 180 degrees to face forward and bend elbows until forearms are perpendicular to body, keeping elbows in place. *Simultaneously,* shift weight to right foot, lift left foot slightly off pool bottom, heel first, then toes, and move left foot hip width from right foot.

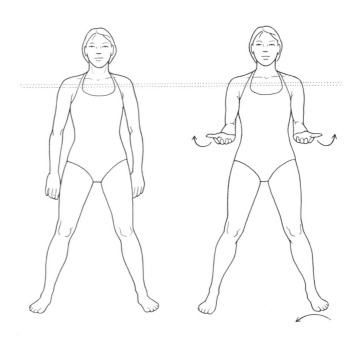

2. As you exhale, touch left toes to pool bottom, lower left heel, and distribute weight evenly over both feet. *Simultaneously,* rotate palms 180 degrees to face downward and return arms to side by straightening elbows.

3. As you inhale, rotate palms 180 degrees so that palms are facing away from body and bend elbows until forearms are perpendicular to body, keeping elbows in place. *Simultaneously,* shift weight to left foot, lift right foot slightly off pool bottom, heel first, then toes, and move right foot to approximately 2 feet from left foot.

4. As you exhale, touch right toes to pool bottom, lower right heel, and distribute weight evenly over both feet. *Simultaneously,* rotate palms 180 degrees to face downward and return arms to starting position by straightening elbows.

5. Repeat 8–10 times.

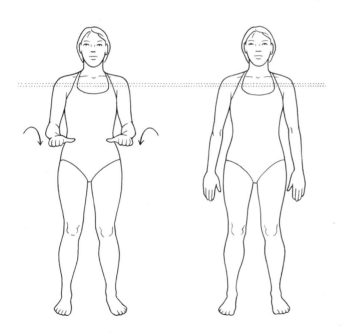

30-MINUTE AQUA FIT WATER TAI CHI WORKOUT

Warm-up ≈ **5 minutes**	Tai Chi Walk Forward Tai Chi Walk Backward

Water Tai Chi Workout
≈ **20 minutes**
(2 minutes each)
	Exercises
	    Tai Chi Opening
	    Circle Water Spray Right (4 times)
	    Circle Water Spray Left (4 times)
	    Roll the Ball
	    Hands Like Clouds
	    Yin Yang
	    Full Moon
	    Tai Chi Closing

Relaxation ≈ **5 minutes**	Calming Breath (8–10 times) Rhythmic Breath (8–10 times)

CHAPTER FIVE

"SPAAAH" RELAXATION

People began using the word "spa" to describe popular mineral springs in Spa, Belgium. In this section, I use the word "spa" more generally, referring to any warm-water bath.

Recall that aquatic environments increase circulation, bringing more oxygen and nutrients to muscles, tendons, and ligaments, as well as carrying away the by-products of inflammation. Warm spa water increases circulation even more than pool water. Furthermore, the oxygen cost of breathing is lower at higher temperatures, so that more oxygen is shunted to muscles. For these reasons, spas are an excellent tool for the treatment of injuries and inflammation.

In addition, many spas, often called whirlpools, have massaging jets. Jet water pressure further increases circulation to the body part at which it is directed. In cases of inflammation or injury, alternating five minutes of jet massage or warm spa water with five minutes of ice therapy can further increase circulation and promote healing.

Warm water is also sedating and soothing, promoting relaxation and relieving tension. Jets can be used to massage the back or any other body part, increasing relaxation and making spas an excellent tool for relieving stress. Steam clears sinuses and helps respiratory difficulties, and heat increases perspiration to help rid the body of toxins.

Although spas have many extraordinary health benefits, it is very important to observe safety precautions while using a spa. First, always check with your doctor before using a spa, especially if you have heart disease, hypertension, diabetes, kidney disease, or chronic skin problems. Spas are not recommended within the first forty-eight hours after an injury, when ice is more helpful, and if you are pregnant.

Once you get your doctor's approval, never use a spa alone, after drinking alcohol, or for more than fifteen minutes at a time. If you wish to remain in a spa for longer than fifteen minutes, lower the water temperature below 98°F or leave the spa, take a shower, cool down, and return. Pregnant women should use *only* spas that are kept below 98°F, because the mother's environment affects fetal body temperature. Children also should use *only* spas that are kept below 98°F.

Be sure to remove any metal jewelry or watches before entering a spa, as they may otherwise become uncomfortably hot. Always keep a water bottle nearby to prevent dehydration and replace the water that you will lose through increased perspiration. Finally, if you become dizzy or light-headed at any point, exit the spa immediately.

Spas are also not safe for vigorous exercise or immediately following vigorous exercise. However, spas can be an ideal setting for gentle stretches or movements. In fact, in many cases of extreme muscle tension and pain or restricted range of motion, spas are the only comfortable medium for rehabilitation. Stretching and gentle movements in a spa can also help to augment the natural relaxation afforded by warm water.

The following section contains step-by-step how-to instructions for the gentle stretches below, which combine yoga asanas, water rehabilitation, and traditional stretches. So relax and melt away the stress. Begin by seating yourself comfortably in a spa, give yourself a back massage with whirlpool jets, and treat yourself to "spaaah" relaxation.

- Foot Massage
- Hand Massage
- Shoulder Shrugs
- Seated Forward Bend
- Hip Hugs

- Diamond Asana
- Neck Rolls
- Spa Mermaid/Merman
- Aqua Arms

FOOT MASSAGE

Massages and relaxes feet

Helps relieve soreness and pain in feet and ankles

Rx: Arthritis, seniors, running, tennis, sports aches

STEPS

1. If you have access to a whirlpool, try Foot Massage with massaging jets directed at feet.
2. Try these movements actively, without touching feet, or passively, using your hands to move your feet and toes.
3. Simultaneously rotate ankles clockwise 5 times.
4. Simultaneously rotate ankles counterclockwise 5 times.
5. Alternately point and flex both feet 5 times.
6. Wiggle all of your toes as you take 5 deep, full breaths.

HAND MASSAGE

Massages and relaxes hands

Helps relieve soreness and pain in hands and wrists

Rx: Arthritis, seniors, cycling, tennis, golf

STEPS

1. If you have access to a whirlpool, try Hand Massage with massaging jets directed at hands.
2. Simultaneously rotate wrists clockwise 5 times.
3. Simultaneously rotate wrists counterclockwise 5 times.
4. Alternately flex fingers and make loose fists 5 times.
5. Wiggle all of your fingers as you take 5 deep, full breaths.

AQUA FIT TIP ~ *You can do this exercise anywhere to help with hand or wrist concerns, from the bathtub to a sink or bowl full of warm water.*

SHOULDER SHRUGS

Stretches shoulders

Relieves tension and tenderness in upper back, shoulders, and neck

Strengthens shoulders

Rx: Seniors, arthritis, back concerns, cycling, swimming, golf

STEPS

1. If you have access to a whirlpool, try Shoulder Shrugs with massaging jets directed at shoulders.
2. As you inhale, lift shoulders simultaneously up toward ears.
3. As you exhale, relax shoulders down.
4. As you inhale, lift right shoulder up toward right ear.
5. As you exhale, relax right shoulder down.
6. As you inhale, lift left shoulder up toward left ear.
7. As you exhale, relax left shoulder down.
8. As you inhale, bring both shoulders forward.
9. As you exhale, relax shoulders to neutral.
10. As you inhale, bring both shoulders backward.
11. As you exhale, relax shoulders to neutral.
12. Repeat 3 times.

SEATED FORWARD BEND

Stretches backs and fronts of legs

Helps relieve shin splints

Rx: Running, arthritis, seniors, tennis

STEPS

1. Sit on spa step with back against wall of spa.
2. As you exhale, flex right foot and extend right leg as straight as comfortably possible without rounding back.
3. If desired, use a noodle or hands to pull feet toward body.
4. Hold for 5 deep, full breaths, trying to straighten leg more with each exhalation.
5. As you exhale, point toes.
6. Hold for 5 full breaths, trying to straighten leg more with each exhalation.
7. Relax, bend knee to a comfortable angle, and shake legs gently.
8. Repeat on left side.

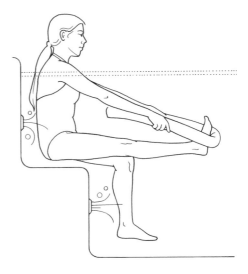

HIP HUGS

Stretches hips and thighs

Rx: Running, tennis, cycling, swimming, seniors, arthritis, back concerns

STEPS

1. Sit with left leg extended, right leg crossed over left leg, and sole of right foot on spa bottom.
2. Grasp lower right leg with both arms and slowly pull toward chest.
3. Hold for 3–5 breaths.
4. Switch legs and repeat.

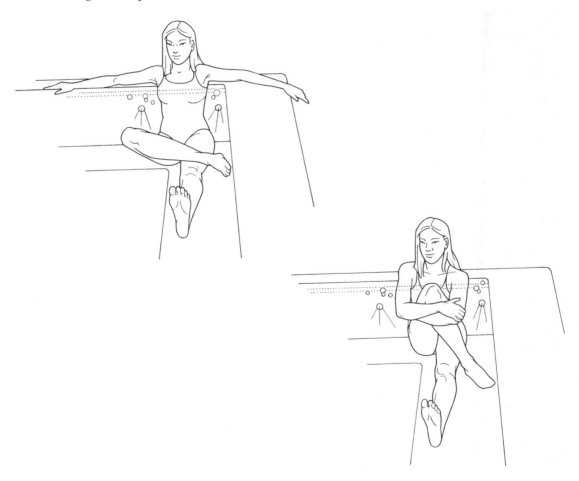

DIAMOND ASANA

Stretches inner thighs

Rx: Seniors, arthritis, tennis, running, cycling, swimming

STEPS

1. Sit with knees bent and the soles of your feet touching.
2. Press knees toward floor with hands.
3. Hold for 5–8 breaths.
4. Switch sides and repeat.

AQUA FIT TIP ~ *Practice Diamond Asana and Hip Hugs consecutively to stretch your inner and outer thighs in balance.*

NECK ROLLS

Relieves neck tension and pain

Stretches neck and shoulders

Rx: Arthritis, golf, tennis, swimming, back concerns, seniors

STEPS

1. If you have access to a whirlpool, try this exercise with massaging jets directed at neck.
2. As you exhale, bring right hand to left side of head and gently pull head toward right shoulder.
3. Inhale and return head to neutral.
4. As you exhale, bring left hand to right side of head and gently pull head toward left shoulder.
5. As you inhale, return to neutral.
6. As you exhale, lower chin to chest.
7. As you inhale, return head to neutral.
8. As you exhale, drop head back.
9. To protect spine in this position, keep shoulders down and back.
10. As you inhale, return to neutral.
11. Repeat 3 times.

AQUA FIT TIP ~ *Alternate using the telephone equally on both sides. Sometimes neck pain results from overusing or favoring one side.*

SPA MERMAID/MERMAN 🤸 🧘

Stretches hips, legs, sides of torso, and chest

Rx: Running, tennis, cycling, swimming, seniors, arthritis, back concerns

STEPS

1. Sit on spa step with legs bent and both feet along left side of hips.
2. Rest left hand on left thigh and right hand on step next to right hip. Use leverage of hands to keep torso squared forward.
3. Bring feet closer to hips for a greater stretch.
4. Hold for 8–10 breaths.
5. Switch sides and repeat.

CHALLENGE: For an added chest and torso stretch, extend arms resting on thigh horizontally and arm resting on floor in an overhead arch.

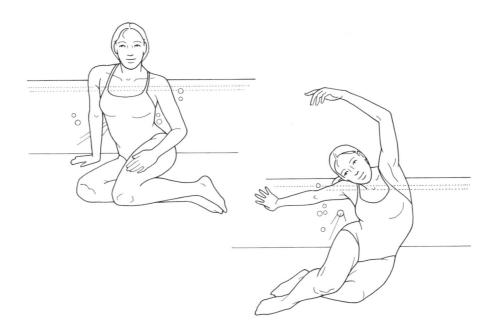

AQUA ARMS

Stretches arms and shoulders

Relieves tension in arms and upper back

Rx: Arthritis, tennis, swimming, golf, cycling, boxing punches

STEPS

1. Extend left arm across chest with thumb upward.
2. Grasp left elbow with right hand and push left arm toward body.
3. Hold for 3–4 breaths.
4. Switch sides and repeat.
5. Raise left arm over head. Grasp left elbow with right hand, bending it and guiding left arm to reach behind head, resting left hand at base of neck.
6. Gently push on the left elbow for additional stretch.
7. Hold for 3–4 breaths.
8. Switch sides and repeat.
9. Extend left arm forward.
10. Pull left fingers toward body with right hand.
11. Hold for 3–4 breaths.
12. Switch sides and repeat.

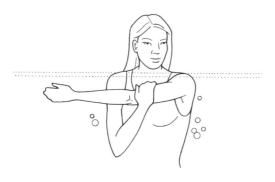
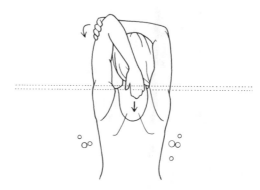

25-MINUTE AQUA FIT "SPAAAH" RELAXATION BREAK

Warm-up ≈ **5 minutes**	Lion (8–10 times) Alternate-Nostril Breath (8–10 times)

"Spaaah"
Relaxation
≈ **15 minutes**
(**1½ minutes**
each)
	Exercises
	    Foot Massage
	    Hand Massage
	    Shoulder Shrugs
	    Seated Forward Bend
	    Hip Hugs
	    Diamond Asana
	    Neck Rolls
	    Spa Mermaid/Merman
	    Aqua Arms

Relaxation ≈ **5 minutes**	Breath Retention (8–10 times) Om Breath (8–10 times)

Warm-up and relaxation should be done in pool, if available.

TRAINING, PRESCRIPTIVE WORKOUTS, AND MORE

Part Two contains exercises and workouts designed to meet your specific needs and lifestyle, whether you are looking for an intense workout, recovering from an injury, or feeling stressed out. A bonus family section for exercisers with young children is also included.

- *Deep-Water Exercises*
- *Sports Cross Training*
- *Prescriptive Workouts*
- *Focused Workouts*
- *Family (Infants, Toddlers, and Children)*

CHAPTER SIX

DEEP-WATER EXERCISES

Deep-water exercise has traditionally been used to stay in shape during physical rehabilitation or after an injury. Professional athletes also use deep-water exercise to complement their training regimes, prevent overuse injuries, and extend their careers. Aqua Fit deep-water exercises are ideal for anyone looking for intense, aerobic, strengthening, no-impact workouts.

Recall that the resistance of water is much greater than that of air. Deep water provides even more resistance than shallow water because more of your body is submerged, helping you build strength and tone muscles. In addition, your feet don't touch the pool bottom in deep water, providing a no-impact workout that doesn't put stress on joints.

The following section details the exercises that make up the foundation of a deep-water workout: jogging/walking, jumping jacks, treading (a safety skill that can also be used as a deep-water exercise), and sit-ups, as well as a special deep-water warm-up exercise and sample workouts that include these skills. Begin all exercises vertically in deep water. For safety and support during deep-water workouts, use a flotation belt or vest. Flotation devices enable you to engage in deep-water workouts and concentrate on form, regardless of your swimming ability. For an added challenge, use hand paddles and/or fins to further increase resistance.

As you begin your Aqua Fit deep-water workouts, remember that they can be vigorous and intense and that experts advise taking it easy when starting a new exercise regimen. According to Judi Sheppard Missett, fitness expert and founder of Jazzercise, it is best to begin an exercise program slowly to avoid injury, burnout, and frustration. Therefore, you may want to try the twenty-minute Aqua Fit deep-water workout before trying any of the longer workouts. Missett also recommends giving up the "all-or-nothing" approach to exercising. Be flexible; listen to your body when you need a day off. Inflexible programs can lead to burnout and injury. Her second bit of advice is to give up the guilt. Stay focused on the day and task at hand; guilt creeps in when you begin regretting the past. Finally, she suggests increasing your exercise by only 5 to 10 percent per week. For instance, if your first week includes two twenty-minute Aqua Fit deep-water workouts, for a total of forty minutes of exercise, increase each workout by only 1 to 2 minutes the following week and continue to increase gradually.

- Ladder Stretch
- Deep-Water Walking
- Deep-Water Jogging
- Deep-Water Treading
- Deep-Water Jumping Jacks
- Deep-Water Sit-ups
  In Shallow Water
  Deep-Water Training Principles

LADDER STRETCH

Stretches calves and hamstrings

Warms up legs for deep-water workout

STARTING POSITION: Stand on tiptoes on bottom rung of ladder, facing pool wall and holding ladder railings for support.

STEPS

1. As you exhale, alternately lower heels below the ladder rung.
2. As you inhale, return to tiptoes.
3. Repeat 10 times.
4. Be sure to maintain a supporting grasp on the rail while doing this exercise. Before beginning, notice if the rail is slippery or easy to hold.

ADJUSTMENT: Pool steps are preferable to a ladder if balance is a concern.

DEEP-WATER WALKING ⊕ ⊛

Aerobic exercise

Strengthens entire body

STARTING POSITION: Assume vertical position in deep water. Your flotation belt will help keep you vertical and supported.

STEPS

1. Walk as if you are on land and you will make slow, steady forward progress.
2. Maintain a vertical posture rather than assuming a horizontal "swimming" posture.
3. Water-walk forward, moving right arm forward with left leg and left arm forward with right leg.
4. Water-walk backward, moving right arm forward as you move left leg backward and left arm forward as you move right leg backward.

CHALLENGES

1. Separate legs farther with each step.
2. Straighten arms and extend them to 45 degrees with each step.

DEEP-WATER JOGGING 🏋 🏃

Aerobic exercise

Strengthens entire body

STARTING POSITION: Assume vertical position in deep water.

STEPS

1. Jog as you do on land.
2. Move right arm forward with left leg and left arm forward with right leg.
3. Lean forward slightly.

ADJUSTMENT: Wear a flotation device. Slice hands through water with thumb leading.

CHALLENGE: Try "running uphill" by decreasing speed, increasing range of motion, and leaning forward. Lift right knee to hip height, then reach out with your right leg, as far as possible, getting full extension similar to a hurdle. Simultaneously extend left leg as far as possible backward. Flatten hands with paddle or mitts for greater resistance.

DEEP-WATER TREADING

Aerobic exercise
Strengthens entire body

STARTING POSITION: Assume vertical position in deep water.

STEPS

1. Use arms in a sculling motion
   and legs in one of many
   motions: bicycling, scissors,
   frog, or whip action.

2. *Sculling:* Start with both arms
   bent to 90 degrees and elbows
   near waist. Create a continuous figure-eight motion with
   both hands, moving them
   simultaneously away from the
   body and back to starting
   position.

3. *Leg motions:* Frog and whip-
   action leg motions are variations on bicycling, with knees
   closer together for whip
   action and farther apart for
   frog. A scissors leg motion
   involves bending both knees
   toward chest, straightening
   legs so that feet are hip width
   or wider apart, and then
   bringing straight legs together.

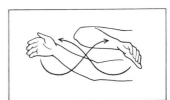

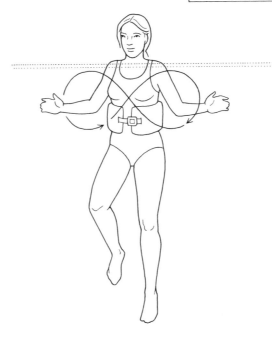

ADJUSTMENT: Wear flotation support.

CHALLENGES

1. Experiment with propelling and stabilizing upper body higher above the water. Try treading with chin, shoulders, or chest in the air.
2. Try treading with your legs only while holding your arms above water.
3. *Tug-of-war:* In chin-deep water, use a reverse scull with palms up as you tread with your legs. The reverse scull will press you underwater, while the treading will keep you up. See which is *your* better half!
4. For more resistance, try sculling with one hand at a time, alternating arms.

DEEP-WATER JUMPING JACKS

Aerobic exercise
Strengthens entire body

STARTING POSITION: Assume vertical position in deep water. Wear flotation belt.

STEPS

1. Begin with hands at sides and legs together.
2. As you exhale, sweep hands to a vertical position in a 180-degree arc and move feet hip width apart.
3. As you inhale, return to starting position.

ADJUSTMENT: Bring hands and arms 45 degrees under surface of water.

CHALLENGES

1. Cross arms and/or legs alternately in front and in vertical position.
2. Hold a kickboard in each hand, with the long axis parallel to and touching each arm or use barbells.

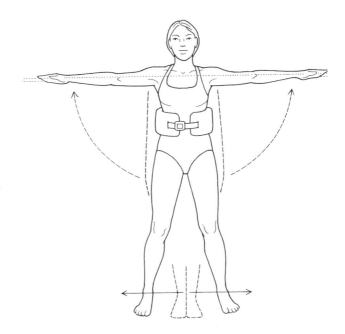

AQUA FIT TIP ~ *Working against the water's buoyancy and resistance as you push your arms and legs back toward your body makes these deep-water jumping jacks a great workout.*

DEEP-WATER SIT-UPS

Strengths abdominal muscles

STARTING POSITION: Assume vertical position in deep water.

STEPS

1. Scull with your arms as if treading to stay vertical and afloat.
2. As you exhale, draw knees toward chest.
3. As you inhale, straighten legs.
4. As you exhale, twist torso and draw knees toward right side.
5. As you inhale, straighten legs.
6. As you exhale, twist torso and draw knees toward left side.

CHALLENGE: For a vigorous sit-up, float on back with knees bent and calves resting on pool deck (or someone holding them). Supporting head with hands, tuck chin up to chest and return to starting position.

ADJUSTMENT: Add a flotation belt or noodle for support and buoyancy.

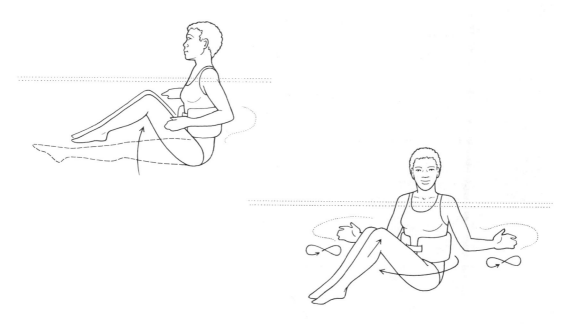

IN SHALLOW WATER

WHY

There are two common reasons for doing deep-water Aqua Fit workouts in the shallow end. First, some pools aren't deep enough for traditional deep-water exercise or to accommodate taller exercisers. Second, some exercisers may not feel comfortable yet in deep water.

HOW

There are many ways you can adapt your deep-water exercise to shallow water.

1. Try deep-water exercise in one of the following horizontal positions by supporting your upper body and simulating any deep-water exercise with your legs. This takes concentration, as you will find that movements such as running, skipping, and hopping are so intuitive that initially you may not be able to replicate them in a horizontal position. However, physically and mentally, it is great exercise to try.
   - In a prone position, support upper body with a kickboard or other flotation device.
   - Hold on to pool edge with arms extended and body floating in a prone position. Use a bracket position for extra support, holding pool edge with one hand and pushing off pool wall with other hand.
   - Float on back, holding pool corner with one arm on each wall.
   - Float on back wearing a flotation belt and support upper body using a noodle behind neck with one end under each arm or with one kickboard under each arm at sides.
2. Remain vertical, but use multiple flotation devices to support and position yourself higher in the water. For instance, use a noodle between your legs and a flotation belt.
3. Switch from a vertical stance and lean forward while you are jogging, so that while more of your body is submerged, your feet don't touch the floor of the pool.
4. Add more sit-ups with your calves on the pool deck to your workout. These can be done in water of any depth.

DEEP-WATER TRAINING PRINCIPLES

- **Interval training.** Using a pace clock or wristwatch, count the number of repetitions you complete or steps you take in a given time period. Rest, repeat, and try to increase the number for the same time period. Try an Aqua Fit breathing exercise while you're resting. Counting your repetitions is a great way to meditate by focusing on your bodily sensations.
- **Fartlek Method.** The Fartlek training method of alternating easy and hard intervals is used by athletes to increase endurance and cardiovascular capacity. Try alternating deep-water jogging or treading with your arms above water with deep-water walking or treading slowly.

20-MINUTE AQUA FIT DEEP-WATER WORKOUT

Warm-up ≈ **5 minutes**	The Hundred Ladder Stretch
Deep-Water Workout ≈ **10 minutes**	Exercises *(1 min.) Walking* *(1 min.) Treading* *(1 min.) Jumping Jacks* *(1 min.) Jogging (easy)* *(30 sec.) Jogging (hard)* *(30 sec.) Jogging (easy)* *(25 sec.) Jogging (hard)* *(25 sec.) Jogging (easy)* *(20 sec.) Jogging (hard)* *(20 sec.) Jogging (easy)* *(15 sec.) Jogging (hard)* *(15 sec.) Jogging (easy)* *(10 sec.) Jogging (hard)* *(10 sec.) Jogging (easy)* *(5 sec.) Jogging (hard)* *(5 sec.) Jogging (easy)* *(1 min.) Sit-ups*
Relaxation ≈ **5 minutes**	Ladder Stretch Rhythmic Breath

30-MINUTE AQUA FIT DEEP-WATER WORKOUT

Warm-up ≈ **5 minutes**	The Hundred Ladder Stretch
Deep-Water Workout ≈ **20 minutes**	Exercises *(4 min.) Walking* *(4 min.) Treading* *(4 min.) Jumping Jacks* *(4 min.) Jogging* *(4 min.) Sit-ups*
Relaxation **5 minutes**	Ladder Stretch Calming Breath (8–10 times)

45-MINUTE AQUA FIT DEEP-WATER WORKOUT

Warm-up ≈ **5 minutes**	The Hundred Ladder Stretch

Deep-Water
Workout
≈ **35 minutes**
	Exercises
	    (2 min.) Walking
	    (2 min.) Jogging
	    (2 min.) Treading (arms and chest above water)
	    (3 min.) Sit-ups (calves on pool deck)
	    (3 min.) Treading (arms and chest above water)
	    (3 min.) Jogging
	    (3 min.) Treading (arms and chest above water)
	    (3 min.) Jumping Jacks (holding 2 kickboards)
	    (45 sec.) Treading (fingers above water)
	    (45 sec.) Treading (right hand above water)
	    (45 sec.) Treading (left hand above water)
	    (45 sec.) Treading (fingers above water)
	    (1 min.) Sit-ups
	    (2 min.) Tug-of-War Treading
	    (1 min.) Sit-ups
	    (1 min.) Jumping Jacks

Relaxation ≈ **5 minutes**	Ladder Stretch Om Breath

CHAPTER SEVEN

SPORTS CROSS TRAINING

Aqua Fit sports cross training includes intense boot camp workouts for runners, racquet sport players, skiers, bikers, triathletes, and golfers, as well as over a dozen other sport-specific exercises to improve technique, a guide to preparing for a triathlon, and a circuit training workout. Aqua Fit sports cross-training workouts build strength and endurance to enhance sports performance, while relaxing and stretching muscles to prevent and rehabilitate injury.

Cross training is a technique used to enhance performance by athletes that entails building fitness that is not specific to their sport. For instance, football, basketball, and soccer players often run and lift weights to increase strength and endurance. Cross training helps prevent repetitive-use injuries that could occur from, say, swinging a bat or throwing a football for too many hours in a row. Therefore, training that is not sport-specific is often used to stay fit during the off-season, prolong careers, and minimize downtime from injury.

Cross-training in water provides athletes with the opportunity to train in a virtually no-impact environment, without shock or strain on joints, which is particularly useful during rehabilitation. In addition, water's substantial and uniform resistance strengthens and tones muscles. Finally, water's air-conditioning effect provides a more comfortable medium than land for working out in hot or humid weather.

In addition to building fitness that is not sport-specific through cross training, aquatic environments are ideal for practicing sport-specific skills. Water slows down motion so that you can concentrate on the techniques of sport-specific movements to improve performance. To use this method, first observe an elite athlete in your sport, isolating techniques that you wish to reinforce. Practice the skill on land, perhaps watching in a mirror so you can see yourself move. Then transfer the skill to water and incorporate it into your Aqua Fit workout. In this manner, you can practice a reverse lay-up, golf swing, or tennis serve in the pool.

In the following section, the basic movements of over a dozen sports have been isolated for a water environment to help teach and reinforce technique, while strengthening and stretching muscles for improved performance. Each exercise includes a starting position, step-by-step how-to instructions, and appropriate challenges or adjustments. Choose a mixture of exercises. The times are approximations. Finally, a fun, stimulating circuit-training workout includes exercises from multiple sports.

It also contains training camp workouts for runners, racquet sport players, skiers, and golfers, which include Aqua Fit water yoga, Pilates, and tai chi, as well as deep-water exercises, in addition to an opportunity to practice sport-specific technique in an aquatic environment. Each workout is designed to enhance performance and help prevent injury through strengthening and stretching specific muscles, as well as build cardiovascular endurance. As with the deep-water workouts in the previous section, these training camp workouts are intense and vigorous, so be sure to start slowly, especially if you are deconditioned, and always listen to your body.

- Boxing Punches
- Basketball
- Downhill Ski Moguls
- Cross-Country Skiing
- Aqua Hurdles
- Sports Swing

- Volleyball
- Soccer Kick
- Mountain Climbing
- Swimming
- Water Dancer

BOXING PUNCHES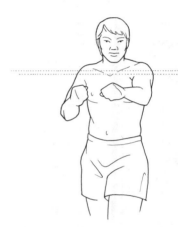

Strengthens arms, shoulders, and chest

STARTING POSITION: Stand in chest-deep water on balls of feet with slight bend in knees, legs hip width apart, and right foot slightly in front of left foot. Make fists with both hands and hold in front of body at chest level.

STEPS: For the following three boxing techniques, extend left arm as you exhale, inhale as you return to starting, and repeat. Next, reverse starting position so that left foot is slightly in front of right foot and repeat all punches with right arm. Keep a bend in punching arm to protect elbow.

1. *Jab:* Punch fist forward from body at chest level.
2. *Hook:* Punch fist across body at chest level.
3. *Undercut:* Punch upward, moving fist from waist level to chest level.

ADJUSTMENT: Practice one technique at a time.

CHALLENGE: Use mitts or gloves for extra resistance.

BASKETBALL

Strengthens legs, arms, shoulders, and front of torso

STARTING POSITION: Stand in shoulder- to chest-deep water.

STEPS: Practice shooting, dribbling, and passing.
1. *Shooting.* Jump as high as possible out of the water as if shooting a basketball. Bend knees and then straighten them as you spring up off both feet. Practice left- and right-handed shooting. Remember to follow through and flick wrist of shooting hand. Use a water basketball setup if available.
2. *Passing.* Practice the motions of chest- and bounce-passing a basketball with both arms underwater. Remember to follow through with both arms after passing.
3. *Dribbling.* Practice dribbling left- and right-handed.

CHALLENGE: Hold pull-buoys or barbells while practicing passing and dribbling for extra resistance.

AQUA FIT TIP ~ *Try using aqua shoes for added traction during basketball, volleyball, cross-country skiing, and soccer Aqua Fit training.*

DOWNHILL SKI MOGULS

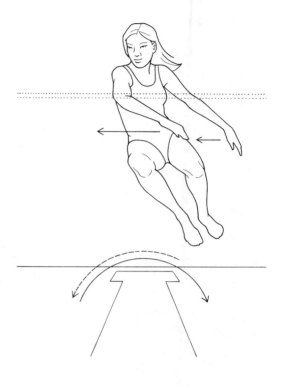

Strengthens entire body

STARTING POSITION: Stand in chest-deep water with feet together next to swim line that marks lap lanes. Use another stationary line or a virtual line on pool bottom if lane line is not available.

STEPS

1. Keeping feet together, jump over line by bending knees and pushing water to opposite side with both hands.
2. Jump back to starting position.

CHALLENGE: Use hand paddles, mitts, or barbells to simulate poles.

CROSS-COUNTRY SKIING 🏋️ 🏃

Strengthens entire body

STARTING POSITION: Stand in chest-deep water with legs shoulder width apart.

STEPS

1. Extend right arm and left leg forward.
2. Then jump and alternate left arm forward and right leg forward.
3. Jump and alternate forward and backward motion, with arms and legs moving in opposition to each other, maintaining equal strides.

CHALLENGE: Use hand paddles, mitts, or barbells to simulate poles for extra resistance.

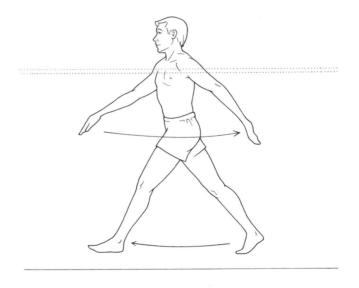

AQUA HURDLES

Strengthens buttocks, quadriceps, and hamstrings

STARTING POSITION: Stand in chest-deep water.

STEPS

1. Begin with knees together under body.
2. Simultaneously extend right leg straight forward and left leg behind you.
3. Return to starting position and repeat with opposite leg forward.

CHALLENGE: Use an aqua step if available (underwater step equipment). Practice clearing the step, first widthwise, then lengthwise.

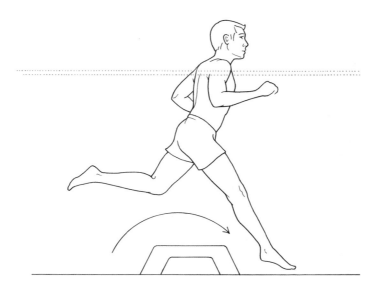

SPORTS SWING

Strengthens sides of torso, abdomen, lower back, arms, and shoulders

STARTING POSITION: Stand in chest-deep water.

STEPS

1. Practice appropriate swing for tennis, golf, baseball, squash, or racquetball.
2. Hold both arms together and swing, paying attention to correct mechanics of chosen sport and remembering to follow through.

CHALLENGE: Hold hand paddles, pull-buoys, or barbells with both hands for added resistance.

VOLLEYBALL 🏋 🏃

Strengthens entire body

STARTING POSITION: Stand in chest-deep water.

STEPS: Practice the motions of spiking, setting, and serving. When setting, jump as high as possible out of the water and remember to pike hips up. Use a real ball if available.

ADJUSTMENT: Practice vertical jumping without arm movements.

CHALLENGE: Wear paddles or mitts while practicing serves for extra resistance.

SOCCER KICK 🏋 🏃

Strengthens legs and hips

STARTING POSITION: Stand in chest-deep water with room to kick legs forward.

STEPS: Practice soccer kicks with both feet. Remember to extend leg forcefully and vary foot position.

ADJUSTMENT: Practice soccer kicks while holding on to the wall.

CHALLENGE: For extra exertion, place a resistance cuff on your ankle.

MOUNTAIN CLIMBING

Strengthens back, arms, shoulders, and legs

STARTING POSITION: Stand at a comfortable depth, facing pool wall and grasping pool edge with both hands.

STEPS
1. Place feet flat on pool wall just above pool floor.
2. Slowly walk up wall, no farther than waist level.
3. Return to a standing position by slowly walking down the pool wall.

ADJUSTMENT: Hold on to the pool edge with both feet flat on the pool wall just above the pool bottom. With feet shoulder width apart, bend and flex your legs.

CHALLENGE: Climb with bigger steps alternately to the right and to the left, changing from wall to bottom simultaneously.

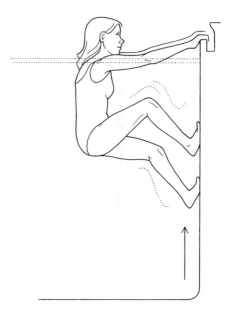

SWIMMING

Strengthens arms, shoulders, legs, abdomen, and upper back

STARTING POSITION: Sit on a kickboard so that your body is mostly submerged but your head is above water.

STEPS

1. Propel yourself forward by stroking with both arms underwater. Practice a dog paddle/crawl stroke motion by alternately stroking forward with both arms.
2. Propel yourself forward again with a breast stroke heart-shaped motion by simultaneously pulling underwater with both arms.
3. Propel yourself backward by reverse sculling with both arms underwater, pushing water forward.

ADJUSTMENT: Practice these strokes while standing, without the challenge of balancing on a kickboard.

CHALLENGE: Wear gloves or use hand paddles for added resistance.

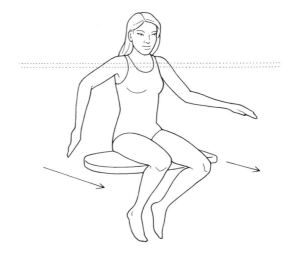

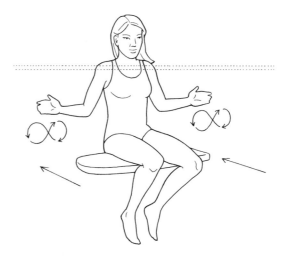

WATER DANCER

Strengthens and stretches entire body

STARTING POSITION: Stand with your feet together in waist- to chin-deep water.

STEPS: Try all of your favorite dance moves in the pool. In water, you'll land safely on your feet even when you try the most outrageous dance moves! You'll also help to tone your muscles gracefully.

AQUA CIRCUIT CROSS-TRAINING WORKOUT

Aquatic circuit cross training combines exercises for many different sports in one workout. Different aquatic equipment for each exercise can also be placed at each station. This workout is most effective when an exerciser or group of exercisers has access to an entire pool or a large part of a pool. Each exerciser begins at one station (i.e., cross-country skiing with aqua barbells), practices for a set period of time (i.e., five minutes), and then moves to the next station (i.e., boxing punches with gloves).

The following aquatic circuit cross-training workout can add some variety and excitement to your exercise routine. In addition, aquatic environments are ideal for beginning to learn new sports, with less risk of falling or injury. The suggested blueprint below can be used to set up the stations for your aqua circuit.

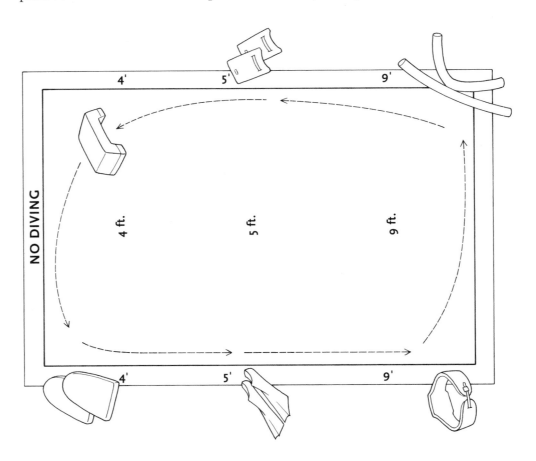

45-MINUTE CIRCUIT CROSS-TRAINING WORKOUT

Warm-up ≈ **5 minutes**	Breath of Fire (5–7 times) Alternate-Nostril Breath (8–10 times)

	Circuit Cross Training		
	Station	*Exercise*	*Suggested Equipment*
Circuit	1	Boxing Punches	Gloves
Cross-Training	2	Basketball	Hand Paddles
Workout	3	Downhill Ski Moguls	Barbells
≈ **35 minutes**	4	Cross-Country Skiing	Barbells
(**3 minutes**	5	Aqua Hurdles	Aqua Step
per station,	6	Sports Swing	Pull-Buoy
½ minute	7	Volleyball	Mitts
to rotate)	8	Soccer Kick	Ankle Cuffs
	9	Mountain Climbing	Pool Edge
	10	Swimming	Kickboard

Relaxation ≈ **5 minutes**	Rolling Down the Wall Om Breath

TRAINING CAMP FOR RUNNERS, JOGGERS, AND WALKERS

Running, jogging, and walking can be jarring on knee and ankle joints, as feet pound the ground with each step. Runners, joggers, and walkers can also develop tight or inflexible thighs and calves, which can lead to injury or discomfort. Common running injuries include shin splints, ankle sprains, and pulls in the groin or hamstring muscles.

Over time, the following intense Aqua Fit Runner Training Camp Workout can help prevent injuries as a complement to land running, jogging, or walking. You can also use it to take a break from high-impact exercise or on a day that's too hot or humid for pounding the pavement. It will help stretch the groin, hamstrings, and calves, as well as build cardiovascular capacity.

45-minute Runner Training Camp Workout

Warm-up ≈ **5 minutes**	Lion (8–10 times) Sun Salutations (4 times)

Runner's
Training Camp
Workout
≈ **35 minutes**
(**1½ minutes each**
if not noted)
	Water Tai Chi
	    Circle Water Spray Right
	    Circle Water Spray Left
	Water Yoga
	    Downward Dog
	    Warrior
	    Toe Lock
	    Chest Expansion
	    Mountain
	Deep-Water Exercises
	    (4 min.) Jogging
	    (2 min.) Treading (arms and chest above water)
	    (4 min.) Jogging
	    (2 min.) Treading (arms and chest above water)
	    (3 min.) Walking
	Water Pilates
	    Ballet Legs
	    Scissors
	    Corkscrew
	    Leg Crossover
	    Clam

Relaxation ≈ **5 minutes**	Breath Retention (8–10 times) Rhythmic Breath (8–10 times)

TRAINING CAMP FOR TENNIS, SQUASH, AND RACQUETBALL PLAYERS

Tennis, squash, and racquetball are vigorous sports that can take a toll on the body. The high impact of the feet hitting the court can be jarring on joints. In addition, the torque of side-to-side movements can twist or put pressure on knees and ankles, as well as pull groin muscles. For these reasons, groin, ankle, and knee injuries are common among racquet sport players. Reaching with a racquet can put strain on shoulders, as can repetitive swinging on elbows. Hence, shoulder injuries and tennis elbow are also common among racquet sport players.

The following Aqua Fit Racquet Sports Training Camp Workout will help to prevent injury while building skill and technique. It will stretch ankles, inner thighs, groin muscles, arms, and shoulders, as well as increase shoulder range of motion and strengthen knees. Over time, regularly incorporating Aqua Fit cross training into your fitness routine will extend your racquet sport playing years.

45-MINUTE RACQUET SPORTS TRAINING CAMP WORKOUT

Warm-up ≈ **5 minutes**	Sun Salutations Breath of Fire

Racquet Sports
Training Camp
Workout
≈ **35 minutes**
(**1½ minutes each
if not noted**)
	Cross Training
	    (4 min.) Sports Swing
	Water Tai Chi
	    Roll the Ball
	    Hands Like Clouds
	    Yin Yang
	    Full Moon
	Water Yoga
	    Downward Dog
	    Warrior
	    Shark Circle
	Deep-Water Exercises
	    (4 min.) Jogging
	    (2 min.) Treading (arms and chest above water)
	    (4 min.) Jogging
	    (2 min.) Treading (arms and chest above water)
	    (3 min.) Walking
	Water Pilates
	    Scissors
	    Leg Crossover

Relaxation ≈ **5 minutes**	Om Breath Calming Breath

TRAINING CAMP FOR GOLFERS

The sport of golf is both physically and mentally demanding. Over time, practicing the Aqua Fit water tai chi exercises in the following Golfer Training Camp Workout can improve your concentration and performance, helping you stay focused and centered throughout your round.

In addition, this workout will stretch the sides of your torso, spine, wrists, and arms, increasing your range of motion, lateral flexibility, and swing control. Finally, practicing your swing in an aquatic environment will improve your technique. Aqua Fit cross training for golf is the brand-new approach that you've been looking for to shave strokes off your score.

45-MINUTE GOLFER TRAINING CAMP WORKOUT

Warm-up ≈ **5 minutes**	Tai Chi Walk Forward Tai Chi Walk Backward

Golfer's
Training Camp
Workout
≈ **35 minutes**
(**1½ minutes each**
if not noted)
	Cross Training
	  (5 min.) Sports Swing
	Water Tai Chi
	  Tai Chi Opening
	  Circle Water Spray Right
	  Circle Water Spray Left
	  Roll the Ball
	  Hands Like Clouds
	  Yin Yang
	  Full Moon
	  Tai Chi Closing
	Water Yoga
	  Upward Dog
	  Aqua Lunge
	  Shark Circle
	  Water Wheel
	  Mountain
	Water Pilates
	  Leg Kicks
	  Spinal Twist
	  Mermaid/Merman
	  Clam
	Cross Training
	  (3 min.) Sports Swing

Relaxation ≈ **5 minutes**	Om Breath Calming Breath

TRAINING CAMP FOR CYCLISTS

Besides injuries caused by falls, the most common afflictions among cyclists are back problems, which can be caused by imbalances in strength between the abdominal and back muscles. The first line of defense against such back pain is attention to posture while riding. It is important to keep shoulders down and back and avoid rounding over the handlebars.

Over time, the Aqua Fit exercises in the following Cyclist Training Camp Workout will help stretch your abdominal and chest muscles, while strengthening your upper and lower back to correct postural imbalances and prevent back pain. The workout will also improve overall flexibility, which helps prevent injuries during falls. Finally, Aqua Fit cross training will enhance your performance by increasing cardiovascular capacity and strengthening leg muscles.

45-MINUTE CYCLIST TRAINING CAMP WORKOUT

Warm-up ≈ **5 minutes**	The Hundred Breath of Fire

Cyclist
Training Camp
Workout
≈ **35 minutes**
(**1½ minutes each
if not noted**)
	Water Yoga
	    Mountain
	    Upward Dog
	    Plank
	    Shark Circle
	    Chest Expansion
	    Water Wheel
	Deep-Water Exercises
	    (2 min.) Jogging
	    (4 min.) Treading (legs in bicycle motion)
	    (2 min.) Jogging
	    (4 min.) Treading (legs in bicycle motion)
	    (3 min.) Walking
	Water Pilates
	    Leg Circles
	    Tub Turn
	    Scissors
	    Mermaid/Merman
	    Leg Kicks
	    Single Leg Stretch

Relaxation **5 minutes**	Back Float Calming Breath

TRAINING CAMP FOR SWIMMERS

Swimming is a total-body workout that requires a total-body strengthening and stretching cross-training workout. The most common complaints among swimmers are lower back pain and shoulder injuries. Lower back pain in swimmers can be caused by an imbalance in strength between the front of the torso, upper back, and lower back.

The following Aqua Fit workout will stretch and strengthen the entire body with a focus on stretching the shoulders, ribs, and upper back while strengthening the lower back and increasing shoulder range of motion. At the same time, the swimming cross-training exercise is a very useful tool for focusing on stroke technique and enhancing performance. Finally, the Swimmer Training Camp Workout is a great way to get an intense cardiovascular workout while adding variety to your lap swimming routine.

45-MINUTE SWIMMER TRAINING CAMP WORKOUT

Warm-up ≈ **5 minutes**	Tai Chi Walk Forward Rhythmic Breath

Swimmer's Training Camp Workout
≈ **35 minutes**
(1½ minutes each if not noted)
	Cross Training
	    (3 min.) Swimming
	Deep-Water Exercises
	    (3 min.) Jogging
	    (2 min.) Treading (chest and arms above water)
	    (4 min.) Jogging
	    (2 min.) Treading (chest and arms above water)
	    (2 min.) Walking
	Water Yoga
	    Toe Lock
	    Downward Dog
	Water Pilates
	    Leg Kicks
	    Spinal Twist
	Water Tai Chi
	    Hands Like Clouds
	    Full Moon
	    Yin Yang
	Cross Training
	    (3 min.) Swimming

Relaxation **5 minutes**	Calming Breath Rhythmic Breath

TRAINING CAMP FOR TRIATHLETES

A triathlon is an athletic competition with running, cycling, and swimming components. Triathlon distances vary, from local mini-triathlons to the Ironman, a triathlon held every year in Hawaii, including a 2.4-mile swim in open water, cycling 112 miles over rough terrain, and running a marathon.

Many athletes interested in triathlons have experience biking and running but are new to swimming. The following section includes a few new Aqua Fit exercises that will help you begin to learn swimming skills, along with an overall Triathlon Preparation Workout. This workout will help you learn pre-swimming skills and increase total fitness in preparation for triathlon training. (You can find a comprehensive learn-to-swim program in *Swimming for Total Fitness.*)

Training for a triathlon takes hard work and dedication. In addition, injuries can impede progress if athletes neglect to incorporate stretching into their training regimes. The second workout in this section, the Aqua Fit Triathlete Training Camp Workout, will help stretch and strengthen your entire body. Alternating this workout with your running, cycling, and running workouts can help to keep you limber and injury-free during the grueling training process. The Triathlete Training Camp Workout will also help build total body strength and endurance while adding variety to your exercise program. (If you are only looking to add stretching to your regime or after a workout, try the 30-minute Aqua Fit Flexibility Workout, page 166.)

RIPPLE BREATH

Pre-swimming breathing skill

STARTING POSITION: Standing in chin-deep water, press back, head, buttocks, and heels against pool wall.

STEPS

1. Exhale through the nose and mouth in a steady and deliberate flow as if pushing a small sailboat away from your mouth, creating ripples on the surface of the water.
2. Inhale deeply through the nose and mouth.
3. Repeat 10–15 times.

ADJUSTMENT: Hold on to pool edge with one or both hands.

CHALLENGE: Hold a kickboard just under water surface. As you exhale, blow water off the kickboard.

SPLASH BACK 🏋 🏃

Pre-swimming stroke skill
Strengthens upper back, chest, arms, and shoulders

STARTING POSITION: Stand in chest-deep water.

STEPS: Walk in chest-deep water with crawl arm stroke and splash water backward forcefully as you finish the pull of each crawl arm stroke. The crawl stroke can be divided into three parts: the catch, the pull, and the recovery.

1. *The catch.* Straighten your arm at the elbow, keeping hand relaxed, palm turned slightly outward, and thumb down.

2. *The pull.* With fingers pointed downward, push water straight downward and backward, brushing past your thigh with your thumb. This is the power phase of the stroke.

3. *The recovery.* Bend elbow and lift hand out of water. As you reach forward, turn palm slightly outward with thumb down. Glide hand into water in front of body.

ADJUSTMENT: Practice Splash Back holding a kickboard with one hand and splashing back with the other.

CHALLENGE: Use aqua barbells, hand paddles, or mitts for added resistance.

PILATES SWIMMING

Pre-swimming coordination skill

Strengthens arms, legs, and entire back

STARTING POSITION: Float in a prone position with one noodle under chest and another under pelvis. Or you can float on a raft made by taping two noodles together into a circle.

STEPS

1. As you inhale, simultaneously raise head, right arm, and left leg.
2. As you exhale, return to starting position.
3. As you inhale again, simultaneously raise head, left arm, and right leg.
4. As you exhale, return to starting position.
5. Repeat.

AQUA FIT TIP ~ *Pilates Swimming is a Pilates exercise with the added challenge of balancing on flotation devices in the water.*

FLUTTER KICKS

Pre-swimming kicking skill

Strengthens entire body

STARTING POSITION: Assume a vertical position in deep water, wearing a flotation belt for extra support.

STEPS

1. Move legs back and forth in a continuous, alternating movement with the power originating from the hip and thigh muscles. Your knees should be slightly flexed. Keep your ankles loose and your feet turned slightly inward with big toes brushing in passing.
2. Alternately move straight arms back and forth, while kicking.

ADJUSTMENT: Only move legs. If desired, hold on to two kickboards with arms for extra support.

CHALLENGES

1. Add fins for added resistance.
2. Practice flutter kicks in a horizontal position by holding pool edge or a kickboard.

VIRTUAL STROKE MEDLEY FOR SWIM SKILLS

Arm stroke movement practice

Strengthens arms, shoulders, chest, and upper back

STARTING POSITION: Begin standing in chest-deep water for all strokes.

STEPS

1. *Crawl.* As you walk or jog forward, use crawl stroke arm motion, alternating hand over hand. When you learn rhythmic breathing, add it to stroke by turning head to one side as opposite arm is extended.
2. *Backstroke.* As you walk backward, use alternate windmill backstroke arm motion.
3. *Breaststroke.* As you walk or jog forward, add heart-shaped arm motion. Pull arms simultaneously underwater for the outward pull and recovery. Add breathing by lifting head at the start of pull to inhale and lowering face into water to exhale tiny bubbles.
4. *Sidestroke.* Walking sideways, pull and press arms using a sidestroke arm motion. Begin with arms extended outward, then bring them together in a prayer position under chest. Simulate picking an apple from a tree and putting it in your other hand.
5. *Butterfly.* As you walk or jog forward, try a circular arm motion. Create large forward arm circles with both arms, hands simultaneously pulling through water.

45-MINUTE TRIATHLON PREPARATION WORKOUT

Warm-up ≈ **5 minutes**	Ripple Breath Breath of Fire (5–7 times)

Triathlon
Preparation
Workout
≈ **35 minutes**
(**1½ minutes each**
if not noted)
	Triathlon Training Preparation
	    (3 min.) Splash Back
	    (3 min.) Pilates Swimming
	    (3 min.) Flutter Kicks
	    (5 min.) Virtual Stroke Medley (1 minute per stroke)
	Deep-Water Exercises
	    (4 min.) Jogging
	    (3 min.) Treading (chest and arms above water)
	    (3 min.) Walking
	Water Yoga (2 min. each)
	    Mountain
	    Warrior
	    Toe Lock
	Water Tai Chi
	    Full Moon
	    Yin Yang
	Cross Training
	    (5 min.) Easy Swimming

Relaxation ≈ **5 minutes**	Om Breath (8–10 times) Rhythmic Breath (8–10 times)

60-MINUTE TRIATHLETE TRAINING CAMP WORKOUT

Warm-up ≈ **10 minutes**	Alternate-Nostril Breath Sun Salutations Tai Chi Walk Forward Tai Chi Walk Backward

Triathlete
Training Camp
Workout
≈ **45 minutes**
(**1½ minutes each
if not noted**)
	Cross Training
	    (5 min.) Swimming
	Deep-Water Exercises
	    (5 min.) Treading (legs in bicycle motion)
	    (6 min.) Jogging
	    (5 min.) Treading (legs in bicycle motion)
	    (3 min.) Walking
	Water Yoga
	    Toe Lock
	    Aqua Lunge
	    Shark Circle
	    Water Wheel
	Water Pilates
	    Ballet Legs
	    Corkscrew
	    Clam
	    Single Leg Stretch
	Water Tai Chi
	    Hands Like Clouds
	    Circle Water Spray Right
	    Circle Water Spray Left
	    Full Moon
	    Yin Yang

Relaxation ≈ **5 minutes**	Rhythmic Breath (8–10 times) Breath Retention (8–10 times)

CHAPTER EIGHT

PRESCRIPTIVE WORKOUTS

This section contains prescriptive Aqua Fit workouts for exercisers at various life stages or with specific health concerns, including pregnant women and seniors, as well as people suffering from asthma, arthritis, and back concerns. For some or all people in these categories, land exercise can be painful, dangerous, or unpleasant. Aqua Fit can enable you to remain active with exercise that builds cardiovascular capacity, flexibility, and strength, while enabling you to relax in an aquatic environment. In addition to Aqua Fit workouts, the following pages contain pertinent information and the specific benefits of Aqua Fit for water exercisers in each of the following categories.

- Pregnancy
- Seniors
- Asthma
- Back Concerns
- Arthritis

AQUA FIT PREGNANCY PRESCRIPTIVE WORKOUT

Pregnancy is a special time of your life, and an expectant mother in good condition is better prepared for the physical demands of labor and delivery. Most obstetricians encourage their patients to begin or maintain a sensible exercise program during pregnancy.

However, you should not begin this or any exercise program without the approval of your doctor, who should be kept apprised of your activity throughout your pregnancy. In addition, if you have a sedentary lifestyle, begin with low-intensity physical activity and advance levels gradually.

The American College of Obstetricians and Gynecologists (ACOG) has developed the following guidelines for exercise safety during pregnancy. Regular exercise (approximately three times weekly) is preferable to intermittent activity. Avoid vigorous exercise in hot, humid weather or when you are running a fever. It is important not to become overheated, because the fetus depends on you to control body temperature. Avoid jerky or bouncy movements. Drink liquids liberally before and after exercise to prevent dehydration. If necessary, interrupt activity to replenish fluids. If you experience any unusual symptoms while exercising, stop activity immediately and consult your physician.

Exercising in water can help you follow these guidelines and has many advantages during pregnancy. The air-conditioning effect of water can help avoid overheating. In addition, water's buoyancy takes the stress off joints, allowing virtually no-impact exercise that isn't jarring. Buoyancy also helps alleviate the pressure of the uterus on the bladder and pelvis. Many pregnant women enjoy the feeling of weightlessness afforded by water, especially during the third trimester. The diuretic and natriuretic effects of water, which help rid the body of excess water and salt, can help maintain proper blood pressure, as well as alleviate edema and stiffness. Pregnant women also produce the hormone relaxin, which helps position the hips and pelvis for childbirth but also loosens all of the other joints, which makes land-based exercise risky but water exercise ideal. Finally, hydrostatic pressure helps improve circulation, which can also reduce edema.

Pregnancy is very demanding on the heart and circulatory system, which can lead to edema, or swelling in the hands, ankles, and feet, as well as fatigue. Cardiovascular exercise helps increase the efficiency of the heart and circulatory system and alleviate these symptoms.

Strengthening your back, shoulder, and abdominal muscles can help you sustain good posture throughout your pregnancy and maintain the correct position of the pelvic girdle in relation to the rest of your body. The pelvic girdle is the bone structure that positions your uterus and acts as a funnel through which your baby travels during a vaginal birth.

The following section introduces two Aqua Fit breathing exercises especially for pregnancy as well as the Aqua Fit Pregnancy Workout, which contains water tai chi, yoga, and Pilates, as well as deep-water exercises. Include the deep-water exercises only if you feel suffficiently energetic, and remember never to exercise to the point of heavy breathing or shortness of breath. Try using kickboards and/or noodles under each arm instead of a flotation belt to stay afloat for deep-water exercise. You can use the breathing exercises throughout your workout whenever you need a break or on land to relax and relieve tension during your everyday life.

Over time, the Aqua Fit pregnancy workout will help you build cardiovascular capacity and strengthen your back, shoulder, and abdominal muscles, as well as stretch your inner thighs and groin. Congratulations on taking a step toward a healthy pregnancy for yourself and your child.

KEGEL

Strengthens pelvic and abdominal muscles

STARTING POSITION: Stand in chest-deep water. Use pool corner for extra support.

STEPS

1. Tighten lower abdominal muscles as you contract pelvic floor and vaginal muscles.
2. Hold the contraction and your breath for 5–10 seconds.
3. Take a full breath.
4. Repeat 5 times.

EFFLEURAGE ⊛

Pregnancy breathing exercise

STARTING POSITION: Stand in pool at any comfortable water depth or float on back.

STEPS

1. Place fingers on navel, pointed slightly downward.
2. Trace a circular design on abdomen with fingertips in a continuous motion as you take 3–5 deep, full breaths.

AQUA FIT TIP ~ *Effleurage is a Lamaze breathing technique. Incorporating it throughout your workout will help develop conditioned relaxation of the abdomen.*

30-MINUTE AQUA FIT PREGNANCY WORKOUT*

Warm-up ≈ **5 minutes**	Tai Chi Walk Forward Tai Chi Walk Backward

Aqua Fit
Pregnancy
Workout
≈ **20 minutes**
(1 minute each;
rest as needed)
	Effleurage
	Water Tai Chi
	    Hands Like Clouds
	    Full Moon
	Effleurage
	Water Pilates
	    Scissors
	    Leg Crossover
	    Leg Kicks
	Effleurage
	Water Yoga
	    Child's Pose
	    Aqua Lunge
	    Cat
	Effleurage
	Deep-Water Exercises (optional)
	    Treading
	    Walking
	    Treading
	Effleurage

Relaxation ≈ **5 minutes**	Kegel Effleurage

* Do not begin this or any exercise program without your doctor's consent. He or she should be kept informed of your physical activity throughout your pregnancy.

AQUA FIT PRESCRIPTIVE SENIORS WORKOUT

Regular exercise may also help to slow or reverse decreases in muscle and bone mass that occur naturally with age, as well as the obesity trend in American seniors. Furthermore, exercising is fun and can be an opportunity to socialize.

However, for many seniors it is difficult to remain active due to chronic pain, injury, limited mobility, or illness. It is also safest for seniors to exercise in a climate-controlled environment. Due to the increased range of motion and the air-conditioning effect that water affords, aquatic exercise may enable many seniors to remain active despite these concerns. In addition, there is no danger of falls or bone fractures while exercising in water.

In fact, senior water exercise benefits are currently the subject of much research. In 2002, I taught a ten-week aquatic fitness program to twenty low-income community seniors at the John Jay College pool. The program had many benefits for seniors, both men and women, including social support, an increased sense of well-being, and pain relief, as well as improved circulation, physical health, and self-confidence.

The June 2002 issue of the *Medical Herald* cited a Japanese study in which women between the ages of sixty-five and seventy were divided into two groups. The control group maintained its usual exercise habits. The second group took part in a twelve-week exercise program calling for seventy minutes of water fitness a week, including stretching, warm-ups, endurance, and resistance exercises. Participants in the water fitness program improved their muscle strength and flexibility, as well as lost some fat. The study concluded that water-based exercises can help older women be more independent and perform better with activities of daily living (ADLs).

Water is also an ideal medium for practicing ADLs. The following section contains a list of ADLs, along with suggestions for training in water. While some of the movements may seem basic, practicing them in water can help preserve mobility and restore independent living for seniors or anyone else who is becoming less active. The same movements can then be transferred back to land, making everyday activities easier.

The following section also contains a complete Aqua Fit Senior Workout, which includes water yoga, tai chi, and Pilates, as well as spa and breathing exercises. If balance is an issue or for extra support, stay close to the edge of the pool, hold a kickboard at the water's surface in each hand, hold on to the edge of the pool, and/or wear water shoes. Over time, incorporating this workout into your routine a few times a week will build cardiovascular capacity and gently yet effectively strengthen and stretch your entire body. You can use the Aqua Fit program as an opportunity to play your favorite music and bond with other people your age.

A healthy and fit lifestyle can begin at any age; it's never too late to start. After teaching aquatics for forty years, I still maintain that middle age will always be ten years older than my age, and that water keeps me young at heart!

PRACTICING THE ACTIVITIES OF DAILY LIVING (ADLs)

- Walking. Focus on posture. Travel in different directions (forward, backward, sideways) and with different-sized steps.
- Climbing stairs. Practice moving up and down stairs using an aquatic step or pool steps.
- Turning the doorknob. Reach forward below water's surface with alternate arms. Close fist and rotate palm upward. Bend elbow and bring arm back toward body.
- Small motor movements. Keep fingers strong and limber by practicing everyday movements. Turn keys, play musical instruments, flex fingers, grasp small objects, write your name, dial important phone numbers, use the TV remote, turn the pages of a newspaper or book, or eat with a fork, knife, and spoon. You can also practice these movements in your kitchen sink or tub.
- Dressing. Pass a kickboard from left to right and from back to front. Act as if putting on slacks or a skirt by lifting one leg at a time as high as possible. Put on socks or stockings by bringing one or both hands to alternately raised feet.
- Cooking. Cross arms in front of body underwater and rotate forearms (as if kneading). Then add a grasping motion with your hands, as if picking up a pot. Use gloves or a pretzel made out of a noodle for added resistance.

30-MINUTE AQUA FIT SENIOR WORKOUT

Warm-up ≈ **5 minutes**	Tai Chi Walk Forward Tai Chi Walk Backward

Aqua Fit
Senior
Workout
≈ **20 minutes**
(1½ minutes
each)
	"Spaaah" Relaxation
	    Foot Massage
	    Hand Massage
	    Shoulder Shrugs
	    Neck Rolls
	Water Tai Chi
	    Circle Water Spray Right
	    Circle Water Spray Left
	    Roll the Ball
	    Yin Yang
	Water Pilates
	    Single Leg Stretch
	    Leg Circles
	Water Yoga
	    Mountain
	    Cat

Relaxation ≈ **5 minutes**	Rhythmic Breathing (8–10 times) Rolling Down the Wall

AQUA FIT PRESCRIPTIVE ASTHMA WORKOUT

The most frequent cause of asthma is allergic reaction from dust, animal dander, or some foods. Water exercise is helpful for people with allergy-induced asthma because allergens are usually less prevalent at the water's surface.

In other cases, energetic exercise of five to eight minutes in length brings on an asthma attack. This condition is known as exercise-induced asthma (EIA) and is not the same condition as asthma. Humidity and temperature changes are important factors in inducing asthma during strenuous exercise. Water exercise can improve EIA because water exercisers can more easily maintain a lower core body temperature.

No matter which type of asthma you have, you should take certain precautions while exercising in the water. An inhaler or medication should be brought poolside. Instructors and/or lifeguards should be told about swimmers with asthma. Those with exercise EIA should warm up for ten to fifteen minutes before strenuous activity and alternate five minutes of vigorous activity with five minutes of rest. If an attack occurs, the exerciser should stop immediately and receive appropriate care. Finally, certain ventilation systems in indoor pools retain a high level of chlorine and other pollutants. These may make asthmatic individuals prone to having an attack.

In general, asthmatics should not try to control the pace of breathing or hold their breath. It is advisable that asthmatics should skip certain Aqua Fit breathing exercises: The Hundred, Breath of Fire, Calming Breath, and Breath Retention. However, the combination of rhythmic breathing and movement provided by all other Aqua Fit exercises can be particularly helpful to asthmatics. The following Aqua Fit workout will enable people with asthma to follow these guidelines while strengthening and stretching the entire body, increasing cardiovascular capacity, and relieving stress.

For those needing medication, please consult with your health care practitioner to obtain the appropriate medication prescription prior to exercise.

30-MINUTE AQUA FIT ASTHMA WORKOUT

Warm-up ≈ **5 minutes**	Lion Alternate-Nostril Breath

Aqua Fit
Asthma
Workout
≈ **20 minutes**
(1½ minutes each;
rest as needed)
	Deep-Water Exercises
	    (3 min.) Walking
	    (3 min.) Jogging, easy
	Water Yoga
	    Mountain
	    Warrior
	    Chest Expansion
	    Toe Lock
	Deep-Water Exercises
	    (3 min.) Walking
	    (3 min.) Jogging
	Water Pilates
	    Mermaid/Merman
	    Single Leg Stretch

Relaxation ≈ **5 minutes**	Om Breath Rhythmic Breath

AQUA FIT TIP ~ *Remember to place your "pump" poolside. Rest as needed.*

AQUA FIT PRESCRIPTIVE WORKOUT FOR BACK CONCERNS

Most people will experience back pain or injury at some point in their life. The most simple advice at the onset of back pain of any kind is not to ignore the pain, as people often do. Mild activity is preferable to bed rest; however, you *should* immediately stop doing whatever triggered the pain. Also, applying ice every hour for five to ten minutes can be helpful during the first forty-eight hours after an injury. After two days, heat therapy is helpful for back injuries.

Lower back pain can result from heavy lifting, prolonged bending, excess abdominal weight, poor posture, or muscular imbalances. To prevent back pain from heavy lifting, try not to lean forward while carrying weighty loads. To lower the body for picking up and putting down a large object, bend from the knees, not the waist.

Back pain from excessive bending can be deterred by not assuming any one back position, such as bending over a garden, for prolonged periods. If you are engaging in such an activity, take breaks to stretch and vary back movements.

Finally, to help avoid the lower back pain caused by excess abdominal weight and or poor posture involving a hypercurved lower spine, think about pulling your belly button into your torso and toward your spine. Poor posture or excess weight that leads to a curved lower spine also results in weak abdominal muscles that are out of balance with lower back muscles. This weakness leads to compensation by other body muscles during everyday movements, which leads to more abdominal muscle weakness in a vicious cycle. Strengthening your abdominal muscles and making a conscious effort to improve posture can help to ameliorate these problems.

Upper back pain is often the result of poor posture, such as while sitting at a desk or computer for extended lengths of time. Sitting hunched over a desk can cause tightness in the chest muscles and weak upper back muscles. If you engage in such activity, try to keep the shoulders down and back, and the upper back and neck erect. Arrange your workstation so that you don't have to look up or down at a computer monitor or slouch over a desk that is too low. In addition, take periodic stretch breaks. Try extending both arms sideways and backward as far as comfortably possible, squeezing the shoulder blades together, and dropping the head backward to stretch the chest, strengthen the upper back, and invigorate.

The following Aqua Fit workout provides balanced strengthening and stretching to realign and stabilize your spine. It will help to balance the muscles of the abdomen and chest with the muscles of the back through integrated movements that require the coordination of two or more muscle groups. You can use this workout to rehabilitate injury and relieve pain as well as prevent future back discomfort.

30-MINUTE AQUA FIT BACK CONCERNS WORKOUT

Warm-up ≈ **5 minutes**	Breath of Fire Sun Salutations

Aqua Fit
Back Concerns
Workout
≈ **20 minutes**
(**1½ minutes**
each; rest as
needed)
	Water Pilates
	   Leg Circles
	   Ballet Legs
	   Tub Turn
	   Corkscrew
	   Leg Crossover
	   Single Leg Stretch
	Water Yoga
	   Child's Pose
	   Toe Lock
	   Cat
	   Chest Expansion
	   Mountain

Relaxation ≈ **5 minutes**	Om Breath Rolling Down the Wall

AQUA FIT PRESCRIPTIVE ARTHRITIS WORKOUT

According to Jane Brody's article in the July 30, 2002, *New York Times,* arthritis is the leading cause of disability in the United States, and the wrong way to respond to the stiffness and pain of arthritis is to stop moving. In fact, she writes that regular moderate exercise is extremely important in treating arthritis. It is also crucial to achieve and maintain a healthy body weight to limit stress on weight-bearing joints, such as knees and hips. Water exercise may be particularly beneficial to retain mobility of arthritic joints and manage body weight through low-impact exercise.

Aquatic facilities sometimes offer exercise classes specifically for people suffering from arthritis. Contact your local branch of the Arthritis Foundation for more information.

The following section contains an Aqua Fit workout and the Kickboard Press exercise for exercisers suffering from arthritis in the hands or wrists. The aim of this section is to increase mobility and motor movement while in the water and then transfer that developed flexibility back to land. The water is also an ideal medium for arthritis sufferers to exercise aerobically more comfortably than they can on land. Warm water can be particularly soothing to arthritis sufferers, so look for an aquatic facility with pool water between 83 and 85°F. Over time, the following Aqua Fit Arthritis Workout may help relieve joint pain and inflammation and restore some range of motion, as well as gently build cardiovascular capacity and strength. If you do not have access to a spa, try the spa exercises while seated on a pool step.

AQUA FIT TIP ~ *For joint pain and stiffness in hands and wrists, try submerging hands in a sink or bucket of warm water while pointing and flexing fingers or squeezing and releasing a sponge.*

KICKBOARD PRESS

Strengthens and stretches wrists, fingers, and arms

STARTING POSITION: Stand in chest-deep water, holding a kickboard with curved edge upward behind body. Face elbows outward and hold board close to body.

STEPS

1. Extend arms downward, pressing the board downward as far as possible against the buoyancy of the water.
2. Bend elbows slowly to return the board back to starting position, being careful to control the kickboard.

VARIATIONS

- Press kickboard underwater and return it to the water's surface slowly with your fingertips.
- Hold on to both ends of a kickboard, press the board underwater, and lift the board above the water's surface, creating a waterfall.
- *Isometric push-ups with partner.* With the kickboard held widthwise between two people, one partner presses down while the other presses up for isometric (stationary) resistance.

30-MINUTE AQUA FIT ARTHRITIS WORKOUT

Warm-up ≈ **5 minutes**	Tai Chi Walk Forward Tai Chi Walk Backward

Aqua Fit
Arthritis
Workout
≈ **20 minutes**
(**1½ minutes**
each; rest as
needed)
	"Spaaah" Relaxation
	    Foot Massage
	    Hand Massage
	    Hip Hugs
	    Neck Rolls
	Water Tai Chi
	    Hands Like Clouds
	    Yin Yang
	Water Pilates
	    Mermaid/Merman
	    Spinal Twist
	Water Yoga
	    Upward Dog
	    Downward Dog
	Deep Water
	    (2 min.) Jog (easy)

Relaxation ≈ **5 minutes**	Rolling Down the Wall Calming Breath

CHAPTER NINE

FOCUSED WORKOUTS

The following section contains exercises designed to meet your specific needs and lifestyle, whether you are looking to increase cardiovascular capacity, relax, strengthen and tone, or improve flexibility. You may be a regular runner in need of strength training, or maybe you enjoy using the weight machines at the gym but recognize the need for aerobic training. You can choose one workout that works best for you, pick different workouts based on your mood, or alternate two or more workouts to meet multiple needs.

The Aqua Fit Cardio Workout is designed to get your heart and blood pumping. Try this workout if you'd like to add some aerobic activity to your day or want an invigorating, energizing break. Over time, this workout can increase cardiovascular capacity by increasing the efficiency of your heart and lungs. As a complement to a balanced diet, this workout can also help you shed pounds if you are overweight.

The Aqua Fit Strength/Toning Workout contains exercises to strengthen and lengthen all of the muscles in your body for a toned, lean appearance. With regular practice, this workout will also improve posture and prevent injury, as well as help prevent or reverse bone density loss and osteoporosis.

The Aqua Fit Relaxation Workout is the perfect remedy for a busy, stressful life. Try this workout if your breathing is feeling tense or labored, you want to unwind from a hectic day, or you're preparing for a long, rigorous day. With regular practice over time, this workout can help you feel more centered, patient, focused, and able to cope with daily stresses.

The Aqua Fit Flexibility Workout includes exercises to gently stretch your entire body. Flexibility is a critical fitness component that is often neglected. Stretching can help minimize back pain and muscle soreness and prevent injury, as well as improve circulation and posture.

- Cardio/Aerobic
- Strength/Toning
- Relaxation
- Flexibility

30-MINUTE AQUA FIT CARDIO/AEROBIC WORKOUT

Warm-up ≈ **5 minutes**	Lion Sun Salutations

Aqua Fit
Cardio/Aerobic
Workout
≈ **20 minutes**
(**1½ minutes each**
if not noted)
	Water Tai Chi
	    Tai Chi Opening
	    Circle Water Spray Right
	    Circle Water Spray Left
	    Tai Chi Closing
	Water Pilates
	    Ballet Legs
	    Tub Turn
	Deep-Water Exercises
	    (2 min.) Treading
	    (2 min.) Jogging
	    (1 min.) Jumping Jacks
	    (1 min.) Walking
	Water Yoga
	    Shark Circle
	    Water Wheel
	    Cat

Relaxation ≈ **5 minutes**	Rhythmic Breath Rolling Down the Wall

30-MINUTE AQUA FIT STRENGTH/TONING WORKOUT

Warm-up ≈ **5 minutes**	The Hundred Sun Salutations

Aqua Fit Strength
& Toning
Workout
≈ **20 minutes**
(2 minutes each)
	Water Pilates
	    Leg Circles
	    Tub Turn
	    Corkscrew
	    Spinal Twist
	    Clam
	    Leg Kicks
	Water Yoga
	    Upward Dog
	    Downward Dog
	    Plank
	    Toe Lock
	    Water Wheel

Relaxation ≈ **5 minutes**	Om Breath Breath Retention

30-MINUTE AQUA FIT RELAXATION WORKOUT

Warm-up ≈ **5 minutes**	Breath of Fire Alternate-Nostril Breath

Aqua Fit
Relaxation
Workout
≈ **20 minutes**
(2 minutes each)
	"Spaaah" Relaxation
	    Shoulder Shrugs
	    Seated Forward Bend
	    Diamond Asana
	    Aqua Arms
	Water Tai Chi
	    Tai Chi Opening
	    Roll the Ball
	    Full Moon
	    Tai Chi Closing
	Water Yoga
	    Child's Pose
	    Cat
	    Chest Expansion

Relaxation **3–7 minutes**	Back Float

30-MINUTE AQUA FIT FLEXIBILITY WORKOUT

Warm-up ≈ **5 minutes**	Breath of Fire Alternate-Nostril Breath
Aqua Fit Flexibility Workout ≈ **20 minutes** (**1½ minutes** **each**)	Water Tai Chi 　*Circle Water Spray Right* 　*Circle Water Spray Left* 　*Hands Like Clouds* 　*Yin Yang* 　*Full Moon* Water Yoga 　*Mountain* 　*Warrior* 　*Toe Lock* 　*Chest Expansion* Water Pilates 　*Spinal Twist* 　*Mermaid/Merman* 　*Single Leg Stretch*
Relaxation **3–7 minutes**	Rolling Down the Wall Calming Breath

CHAPTER TEN

FAMILY (INFANTS, TODDLERS, AND CHILDREN)

With today's busy lifestyle, a common obstacle to exercise is the desire to spend time with family. However, just because your child is more interested in games than exercising doesn't mean that you can't spend quality time together during your workout. People of all ages can have fun in the water, from five-month-olds to five-year-olds to seniors. In fact, as you plan your next vacation, take into account the possibilities for family bonding and fitness in water, from aquatic centers and pools to lakes and oceans. Family exercise can be a wonderful strategy for spending more time together, and as the saying goes, the family that plays together stays together.

Aqua Fit "Family" contains useful information about introducing youngsters to water and keeping them entertained once they're there. This section has important safety information as well as game suggestions and fun tips for youngsters of every age.

BABIES AND TODDLERS

This section contains some ideas for bathtime and transitioning into the pool for your young infant or toddler's enjoyment. Teaching your child to enjoy the water will start him or her on the road to a lifetime of safety and fitness. You will also aid in the development of your little one's muscular strength, coordination, and balance. In addition, playing in the water together can be a wonderful bonding opportunity for you and your child. And most important, playing in the water is just fun!

Babies and toddlers are receptive to other people's emotions. Your baby will

The Apex Center Aquatics Complex in Arvada, Colorado, is an indoor water park but has the look and feel of a resort. The complex is leading the trend of taking indoor swimming pools to the next level. The 23,500-square-foot area, with five separate components, is a water paradise for children and their parents alike! Visitors can enjoy two 150-foot water slides; a current channel, which is used for games and water exercise; tethered floating logs for climbing and balance games; a water basketball area; water volleyball nets; an indoor water playground; and a lap pool, which is also used for water aerobics. Finally, they can unwind in one of two whirlpool options, including one that is kept slightly cooler so that small children can enjoy it safely. Planning your next vacation around such a complex is a surefire strategy for getting in your Aqua Fit workouts while your children also have a wonderful time.

learn to enjoy the water if he or she senses that *you* are comfortable and confident in and around the water. Children often learn to be afraid of the water by observing a parent's fear. The bottom line is that you want to instill in your child a sense of security and fun in the water. You can do this by continuously maintaining eye contact, smiling, and cuddling your infant or toddler.

Of course, the most important way to help your infant or toddler enjoy the water is to ensure his or her safety. Never leave your baby or young child unattended near any body of water, including the bathtub, even for a moment. Drowning can occur in as little as one inch of water. In addition, to keep your child healthy and warm, use a hat or towel to cover your infant or toddler's head once he or she leaves the water, since most of the body's heat escapes through the head.

WATER PLAY DURING BATH TIME

Bath time is fun! The benefits of water play go beyond just getting your toddler clean. Talk to your baby or toddler while you bathe him. Begin teaching your child the names of body parts as you say what you are washing. Your little one will gain from learning the names of colors and shapes of objects, as well as new words: "empty," "full," "wet," "dry," "warm," "sink," and so on.

When your child is old enough to sit up on his own, he may be ready to graduate from bathing in the baby bathtub to the regular bathtub. If the child seems hesitant, you can put the baby bathtub in the regular tub a few times, letting him or her grow accustomed to the larger space. You can also try placing a plastic lattice laundry basket into the regular bathtub to give your baby the feel of an enclosed space until he or she is more at ease. If your baby protests against shampooing, try rinsing the hair while the child is wearing a sun visor to keep the water and shampoo out of the eyes.

Bath time is ideal for singing songs or reciting nursery rhymes. Try everything from the traditional "This Little Piggy Went to Market" to "Dem Bones" ("the hip-bone is connected to the thighbone," etc.), or my personal favorite, Bobby Darin's "Splish Splash" (that was also my wedding song!). Try singing "Happy Birthday" and pretending to blow out the candles on the surface of the water to practice ripple breathing when you're done! You can also use rotary arm circles along with your child's songs. Think of "Row, Row, Row Your Boat," or encourage your toddler to kick his or her feet along with your favorite song.

Try playing games with your child as you bathe him or her. Babies and toddlers often enjoy a game of Peekaboo or "painting" the tub with soap bubbles. A slightly older child may enjoy putting his or her face in the water with swim goggles and pretending to be a deep-sea diver. Scooping water and catching objects in the tub develop hand-eye coordination.

You can introduce bath toys once your baby is sitting comfortably in the tub. Babies enjoy plastic kitchen items, such as measuring cups and sponges, as well as fish, dolls, and any toys made of material that do not absorb water and become water-logged. You can add to bathtub fun with terry-cloth puppets, both for washing and for make-believe. A homemade puppet made from washcloths sewn together, with space for your fingers, works just fine. Perhaps the puppet can be the "singer" too!

INTO THE POOL

Many parents enroll their babies and toddlers in parent-child classes at local pool facilities. These classes can be a lot of fun and are an ideal situation for enjoying the water, as well as socializing with others in a relaxed environment. When thinking about signing up for such classes, considerations to look for include warm water, expertise of the instructor, changing areas, cleanliness of the facility, and variable pool depth.

At approximately the age of six months, babies develop a breathing reflex by which they automatically hold their breath. By this age a healthy child is old enough to be in a swimming pool safely. However, I don't recommend ever forcing a child to enter a pool or submerge, especially in cases of severe aversion or crying. The best way to help your child enjoy the water and ultimately learn safety and swimming skills is to honor his or her comfort level.

Once in the water you can simulate "swimming" by holding her in a prone position with one of your arms under her shoulders and your other arm under her hips. When holding a baby in a prone position, remember to hold the hips lower than the shoulders, because a baby's head is very large relative to the rest of the body.

Swim diapers are an essential safety consideration; they are important for everyone's safety to prevent contamination by *E. coli* bacteria. Regular diapers are not snug enough to prevent feces from entering the pool. In the event of an "accident" it takes several hours (six to ten, depending on pool size) to "shock" and clean a pool through a special chlorination process for a pool to be safe again. Swim diapers are sometimes available through vending machines selling individual diapers. Remembering to wash *your* hands *in a sink with soap* after changing your baby's diaper (don't wash them in the pool!) is also an important preventative measure against the spread of *E. coli*.

PRESCHOOL CHILDREN

Your child's enjoyment is the primary objective of teaching him to be comfortable in and around the water. It is a great joy to see kids of all ages in the water, laughing, splashing, and squealing with joy. In addition, helping your child to be comfortable in the water is the first step toward teaching him to swim. Finally, with obesity on the rise in American children, it is important to start thinking about your child's fitness. Although fitness may not be the immediate goal of helping your preschool child enjoy the water, a successful introduction to water activities can have a positive impact on your child's physical and emotional health.

An important but often overlooked aspect of helping your preschooler be comfortable in the water is having her introduction take place in a friendly, safe environment. If the pool environment is clean, the depth appropriate for standing, the water temperature comfortable, siblings or friends present, and the teacher someone with whom your child is familiar, your child is much more likely to enjoy the water and learn to swim. Perhaps you can visit a pool before a session of classes begins to help your child adjust ahead of time. If possible, private or semiprivate lessons are also beneficial.

Patience and encouragement will also accelerate preschoolers' comfort and enthusiasm in the water, as well as learning to swim. Praise their accomplishments and comment on their progress. You can always find something positive to remark on, even if it's the effort in trying. Keep in mind that all children will learn to swim at different rates. There is no set age at which a child is ready to learn to swim or put her head under the water. Some children are naturally more comfortable in the water than others. The best way to support your child's learning to swim is to let the child progress at her own pace.

Finally and most important, before your preschooler gets in the water, keep in mind that an individual trained in rescue breathing techniques should always be present. Although many preschoolers wear flotation devices on their upper arms and/or bathing suits with removable inserts while they are learning how to swim, be aware that these flotation devices don't always keep your child completely afloat. They are not a replacement for learning how to swim. In fact, you may choose to pass on flotation devices so that your child does not learn to rely on them. Take your child's input and comfort level in the water into account when making this decision.

Many preschoolers also enjoy inflatable backyard kiddie pools. Remember to empty these pools when they are not in use; turn them on their sides so that they cannot collect rain water that may become a potential drowning risk.

With these safety considerations in mind, it's time to have fun! Preschool children love toys. Try noodles, animal-shaped slides, Wiffle balls, squishy toys, or anything that's soft and floats. Remember, you don't have to spend a lot to have fun. Make an empty plastic bottle, a watering can, or a funnel into a pool toy. In addition, the following pages include some games that preschool-age children can play to learn pre-swimming skills.

AQUA FIT GAMES FOR PRESCHOOLERS

Aqua ABCs. Children can learn their ABCs by "writing" them underwater with arm or leg motions. They can also sing the ABC song or hum the ABCs underwater. Create an educational game!

Kickboarding. Kicking with a kickboard is a fun way to learn pre-swimming kicking skills. Children can hold on to one end of the kickboard while a parent or adult holds the other end, or children can hold the kickboards by themselves and move through the water. They can also learn to put their faces in the water and blow bubbles at the same time.

Birthday Candles. Children can learn pre-swimming breathing skills by simulating blowing out candles on a birthday cake. Have fun! Sing "Happy Birthday" too, or hum it underwater!

Double Dutch Jump Rope. This exercise lets children practice teamwork and sharing while increasing their comfort level in water. Two children face each other, each holding one end of two noodles parallel to each other, and do jumping jacks. Sing along with your favorite jump rope song. For a change of pace, try jogging while alternately moving the noodles back and forth.

SCHOOL-AGE CHILDREN

School-age children will usually show more interest in interacting with their peers than younger children. Look for opportunities for your child to play with friends in the water. Try having your child's birthday party or special event in a swimming pool. A pool party is sure to be a hit for everyone involved. Just be sure that there is a lifeguard present for safety throughout the party. Summer camp is also a terrific place for children to have fun in the water. Many summer programs offer swimming lessons or time for children to keep cool and splash around in the water together. You may want to consider access to aquatic facilities as you choose a summer program for your child.

Many school-age children are also ready to begin learning basic swimming skills, so this may be an ideal age to enroll children in swimming classes or programs. However, they will still probably enjoy games as well. Therefore, the following section contains Aqua Fit games for school-age children with an emphasis on partner and group games.

AQUA FIT GAMES FOR SCHOOL-AGE CHILDREN

Swimming Through Hoops. Use a hula hoop or make circles out of two noodles taped together. Children can swim through to practice being underwater. Try making a tunnel out of more than one!

Theater/Dancing in the Pool. Everyone is a dancer in the pool; give it a try! It's also great fun to sing or hum underwater. Can the children guess the song? Is there a mermaid (or merman) in your pool?

Ring Toss. Try sinking rings or coins to the bottom of the pool and retrieving them. Remember to have your child exhale while underwater (exhale bubbles through the nose and mouth). One can play this game alone or with two or more people. Who got the most rings?

Kickboard Tug-of-War. Children pair up and face their partners by holding on to one end of a kickboard (held lengthwise) and trying to push the other person back a specified distance by kicking.

NOODLING AROUND:
AQUA FIT GAMES FOR CHILDREN OF ALL AGES!

Noodles are colorful, inexpensive, fun, and safe. However, check whether your pool allows noodles before suggesting these games and instruct children on acceptable conduct. Always supervise water play.

1. Tape two noodles together into a hoop. Use them as basketball nets, or as water polo or soccer goals. (They also make a great raft to hang out on.)
2. Two people can hold two noodles overhead lengthwise to play London Bridge. Swim, walk, or run under the arches.
3. Have a relay log race. Each racer has to hold a noodle around a partner's waist. The "train" (with the noodle around his or her waist) jogs while the "engineer" (holding the ends of the noodle behind his or her partner) kicks!

EPILOGUE

If the benefits of water exercise could be captured in a pill, it would be the most widely prescribed drug in the world. Fortunately, we can get all of the benefits of water exercise with Aqua Fit workouts while we achieve the deep relaxation that restores us to calmness and restfulness.

Water is friendly when we empower it to act as a protector. It enables us to expand our horizons and see the world in a new way. We return to terra firma more optimistic, centered, and flexible, which is essential for both physical and mental health.

Whether you are eighteen, eighty, or beyond, remember that (according to my definition) middle age is ten years older than your age. Water is truly the fountain of youth and will help you to maintain that optimistic attitude and feel young at heart. Thank you for sharing your journey to health and my love of water fitness with me.

"Your body works, the water resists, and you relax.
After Aqua Fit, you feel great!"

—Dorit Shoor,
Aqua Fit participant

SURGEON GENERAL'S REPORT

Lack of exercise can be detrimental to your health.

The following section contains resources and tools for designing and scheduling your own Aqua Fit workouts and charting your progress.

DESIGNING YOUR OWN AQUA FIT WORKOUTS

Now it's time to use all of the Aqua Fit exercises that you've learned to design your own Aqua Fit workouts. What kind of exercises will you choose? Water yoga, Pilates, and tai chi? Or "Spaaah" Relaxation, Deep Water, and Cross Training? You can use the comprehensive benefits listed for each exercise to custom-tailor a program to your unique needs.

Use the following pages to design your own Aqua Fit workouts. Then check off two warm-ups, five to twenty-one main-set exercises, and two relaxation exercises. Choose more main-set exercises for a longer workout and fewer for a shorter workout. Eventually you can design dozens of Aqua Fit workouts, keep them in your Aqua Fit swim bag, and choose one that fits your mood each day!

Warm-up Choose 2 ≈ **5 minutes**	❑ Ladder Stretch ❑ Tai Chi Walk Forward ❑ Tai Chi Walk Backward ❑ Sun Salutations (4) ❑ The Hundred ❑ Breath of Fire (5–7 times) ❑ Alternate-Nostril Breath (8–10 times) ❑ Lion (8–10 times)	

Main Aqua Fit Workout Examples **10-min. set:** Choose 10 1 min. per exercise **15-min. set:** Choose 7 1½ min. per exercise **20-min. set:** Choose 10 2 min. per exercise **30-min. set:** Choose 10 3 min. per exercise	*Water Yoga* ❑ Child's Pose ❑ Mountain ❑ Upward Dog ❑ Downward Dog ❑ Plank ❑ Aqua Lunge ❑ Warrior ❑ Toe Lock ❑ Cat ❑ Chest Expansion ❑ Shark Circle ❑ Water Wheel *Water Pilates* ❑ Leg Circles ❑ Ballet Legs ❑ Tub Turn ❑ Scissors ❑ Corkscrew ❑ Spinal Twist ❑ Leg Crossover ❑ Clam ❑ Mermaid/Merman ❑ Leg Kicks ❑ Single Leg Stretch	*Water Tai Chi* ❑ Tai Chi Opening ❑ Circle Water Spray Right ❑ Circle Water Spray Left ❑ Roll the Ball ❑ Hands Like Clouds ❑ Yin Yang ❑ Full Moon ❑ Tai Chi Closing *Deep Water (1½–2 min. each)* ❑ Walking ❑ Jogging ❑ Treading ❑ Jumping Jacks ❑ Sit-ups *"Spaaah" Relaxation* ❑ Foot Massage ❑ Hand Massage ❑ Shoulder Shrugs ❑ Seated Forward Bend ❑ Hip Hugs ❑ Diamond Asana ❑ Neck Rolls ❑ Spa Mermaid/Merman ❑ Aqua Arms

Relaxation
Choose 2
≈ **5 min.**

❑ Rolling Down the Wall
❑ Back Float (2 ½ minutes)
❑ Breath Retention (8–10 times)
❑ Calming Breath (8–10 times)
❑ Rhythmic Breath (8–10 times)
❑ Om Breath (8–10 times)

CHARTING YOUR PROGRESS: PROGRAM LOG

You can use this page to chart your Aqua Fit progress. Photocopy the table on the following page and fill it out. Over time, you'll be able to tell at a glance how your endurance is increasing if your workouts are twice as long and frequent as they were when you began. If you need a change in your workout, you can analyze this chart to add some variety to your workout. For instance, if you can tell from your chart that you've gotten into a "deep-water rut," you can add some cross training. Congratulations on beginning your program. You know that beginning is half the battle. (And remember, the only way to fail now is to stop trying!)

Date/ Day	Warm-ups	Aqua Fit Main Set	Relaxation	Workout Length/ Intensity	Comments (How Am I Doing?) PG: Personal Goal

CHARTING YOUR PROGRESS: FOOD DIARY

Your eating habits are an important part of your Aqua Fit success. You can photocopy the following chart and use it to keep track of your meals as you make an effort to incorporate more fruits, vegetables, and whole grains into your diet. Comment as you wish in the table with regard to portions, calories, and fat grams.

	Breakfast (A.M.)	Lunch (midday)	Dinner (P.M.)	Snacks (A.M. + P.M.)
Monday				
Tuesday				
Wednesday				
Thursday				
Friday				
Saturday				
Sunday				

STOP THE EPIDEMIC

One in every eight women will have breast cancer in her lifetime. These numbers are shocking whether you're a woman or a man concerned about your wife, mother, friends, or sisters. There are many organizations around the country that are working hard to raise funds for breast cancer research. I've been proud to serve as an honorary chair of the Massachusetts Breast Cancer Coalition's "Against the Tide" swim and now walk campaign for over a decade. The organization raises money for breast cancer research through swimming fund-raisers every June and August in Massachusetts. Contact your local health organization to find out how you can get involved in breast cancer research fund-raisers in your area.

SURGEON GENERAL'S REPORT

Lack of exercise can be detrimental to your health.

DR. JANE KATZ is a full professor at the John Jay College of Criminal Justice in the Department of Physical Education and Athletics; she earned her Doctor of Education degree in Gerontology from Columbia University. As one of the nation's leading authorities on aquatics, she has pioneered water fitness for sports training, recreation, therapy, and wellness. Following the tragedy of 9/11, Dr. Katz created a Wellness Spa to help address the physical, emotional, and spiritual needs of CUNY students, staff, and community at John Jay College.

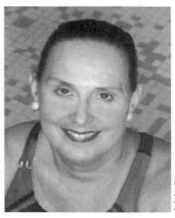
© John Burns

As a member of the 1964 U.S. Synchronized Swimming Performance Team in Tokyo, Dr. Katz helped pioneer the acceptance of synchronized swimming as an Olympic event. Her achievements as a World and National Masters competitive, long-distance, fin swimmer, and synchronized swimmer have earned her All-American and World Masters Championships.

At the 2000 Olympics in Sydney, Australia, Jane Katz was awarded the Federation Internationale de Natation Amateur (FINA) Certificate of Merit to honor her "dedication and contribution to the development" of aquatic sports. She is a member of the Board of Directors of the International Swimming Hall of Fame. While Dr. Katz has navigated swimming pools throughout the United States and beyond, her home pools are all in New York City.

Visit www.globalaquatics.com to learn more and for more information on her instructional video.